STUMBLING THROUGH THE DARK

Thelma Zirkelbach

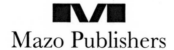

Mazo Publishers

Stumbling Through The Dark

ISBN: 978-1-936778-58-4
Copyright © 2013

The Author
Thelma Zirkelbach
Email: thelmaz@hal-pc.org

Published by
Mazo Publishers
PO Box 10474
Jacksonville, Florida USA 32247

Tel: 1-815-301-3559
Email: mazopublishers@gmail.com
www.mazopublishers.com

Book Production
Prestige Prepress
Email: prestige.prepress@gmail.com

Cover image: Kirill Kurashov | Dreamstime.com

Names of places and people have been changed to insure privacy.

In Memory Of My Husband

ABOUT THE AUTHOR

Thelma Zirkelbach began her writing career as a romance novelist. "Season of Light", written as Lorna Michaels, was the first Harlequin romance featuring a Jewish hero and heroine. The death of her husband in 2005 propelled her from the romance genre to memoir and personal essay. Since then her poems and essays have appeared in numerous journals and anthologies, including Press Pause Moments, This Path, The Poets' Touchstone and Blue Lyra Review.

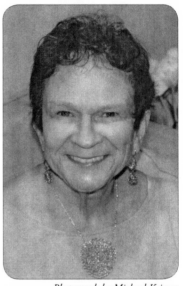

Photograph by Michael Krieger

She recently co-edited the anthology "On Our Own: Widowhood for Smarties". A speech-language pathologist in private practice, she is a graduate of the University of Texas and received her Master's and doctorate from the University of Houston. She is the mother of three and grandmother of two.

A native Texan, she lives in Houston. She blogs at www.widowsphere.blogspot.com

ACKNOWLEDGMENTS

I want to express my thanks to my family and to Ralph's for their love and support for both of us through his illness.

Thanks to my many friends (whose names I have changed) who brought groceries, called, took me to lunch, brought meals, and kept both of us going through our battle.

And a special thanks to the Jewish Chaplaincy Service for their kindness and spiritual support.

Thanks to Gotham Writers Workshop and especially to Ana Maria Spagna, who is an incredible teacher and who saw me through many versions of this manuscript.

To my memoir group from Gotham, Carole Ann Moleti, Reggie LeVerrier, Heather Andersen and Laura Berning, who were part of this journey as I was part of theirs, my thanks for your friendship, input, and support.

And thanks, too, to the Lake Tahoe group, Lyra Halprin, Rossandra White, Tee Graham, and Delphine Boswell, who saw this in its late stages and were generous with encouragement and friendship.

And, of course, to Ana Maria Spagna for instruction and inspiration in Lake Tahoe and to Heather Andersen, who provided the luxurious accommodations there.

To Linda Steinberg, longtime critique partner, thanks for your insight and friendship.

Thanks to Chaim Mazo of Mazo Publishers for believing in this book and bringing it to life.

To Ralph, who faced leukemia with courage and optimism, who loved me in spite of my faults, who made me laugh, who raised my children as his own, who was always there for me, you will forever be in my heart.

To live in this world
You must be able
To do three things:

To love what is mortal,
To hold it

Against your bones knowing
Your own life depends on it;

And when the times comes to let it go,
To let it go.

Mary Oliver,
"In Blackwater Woods"

PROLOGUE

This is my first autumn.

Living all my life in Texas, I've never experienced the change of seasons. Except on calendars, I haven't seen trees clothed in scarlet, coral and gold, colors so brilliant that ordinary words like red, orange, or yellow are too plain for them. I've never crunched fading leaves under my feet or watched the sun set over an autumn landscape. Until now.

Ralph, my husband, often said that nowhere is fall as breathtaking as in his hometown in eastern Iowa. He always wanted me to see the autumn scenery he'd grown up with. Although we visited often in summer and once during a frigid winter, I've never been here at this time of year.

But this isn't the fall I imagined.

Now I'm standing among gravestones, listening to the minister say a final prayer over my husband's coffin, closed forever. A chill late afternoon wind stirs the grass, and I draw my jacket closer around me. My daughter reaches for my hand as we turn away from the grave and trudge back to the car.

I am a romance author. Happy endings are my specialty. I found the hero of my personal love story thirty-five years ago. I'm not supposed to lose him.

I stop and turn to take one more look at the polished wooden casket. Next fall I'll come back, have a headstone placed, and see the leaves again. In this last moment I promise myself and Ralph that I will bear witness to the final year of our life together. I will begin now, while the colors are still fresh; now, before the memories fade like the leaves beneath my feet.

My promise made, I begin a new journey, one I will travel alone.

CHAPTER 1

On Rosh Hashanah the decree is signed, and on the Day of Atonement it is sealed: "Who shall live and who shall die... "

The rabbi spoke the words I'd heard every year of my life, words always spoken on this most solemn day of the Jewish year.

The prayer book depicts God sitting on His judgment seat, with every human soul passing before Him. As each goes by, He inscribes it in one of two books: Life or Death.

In the year 2004, my husband's name was written in the Book of Death.

The last chapter of our story began on the Eve of Yom Kippur, the Day of Atonement. On this night, the Kol Nidre prayer asks God's forgiveness for sins committed in the past year. The congregation stood as organ music resounded through the synagogue and the cantor and choir sang the moving words. The melody filled me with a sense of reverence and peace. It was the last peaceful evening I remember.

When the service ended and we left the sanctuary, Ralph remarked, "I'm getting a sore throat."

Nothing ominous about those words. Fall is allergy season along the Texas Gulf Coast, so I didn't feel the tiniest prickle of apprehension.

I shrugged. "Take some Vitamin C when we get home."

Sometimes events develop so gradually you only notice later that your life has changed. The lines that deepen in your face, the job that no longer challenges, the energy that wanes over time. But those five words uttered by my husband ripped our lives in two. Later, I would think of life until that instant as the Time Before and starting with the next breath, as the Time After.

But that evening when we joined the crowd leaving the synagogue, I was still happy, still secure.

Arm in arm, we walked outside into a September night. The remnants of Hurricane Ivan threatened Texas. Thick, low clouds hid the stars. Rain was forecast for the following morning. I smelled it in the air.

The next day we woke to a gray dawn and the sound of rain drumming on the roof. "I don't want to go to services today," Ralph mumbled.

Although he wasn't Jewish, Ralph always willingly accompanied me to synagogue. I loved Yom Kippur services: the familiar music, the communal confession of sins, the reading from Isaiah. But my throat felt scratchy, too, and in rainy weather the parking lot at our synagogue was often ankle deep in water. I didn't want to get soaked and end up with a sinus infection.

"Maybe we'll go later," I said. Yom Kippur services last all day.

Ralph didn't answer. He'd fallen asleep. When he woke, he asked where I kept the thermometer. His fever was 101 degrees. For the rest of that day and the next he sat around glumly, wrapped in his faded brown bathrobe. Extremely un-Ralph-like.

In the nearly thirty-four years of our marriage, he had the flu once and maybe a couple of sinus infections. He prided himself on his good health and on his ability to "think" himself well if he was feeling under the weather. He even had dental surgery without anesthesia. I always believed it was a rather heroic quality; now I wonder if it was hubris.

On Monday morning Ralph announced he was making a doctor's appointment.

"Make one for me, too," I said. I'd developed an earache.

He scheduled his appointment first.

He phoned after his examination. "Dr. Whitmore says I'm anemic. He said it could be an iron deficiency. The lab's going to run some more tests and he'll call me with the results." He paused. "I'm at Walmart, and you know what? I'm worn out."

"Of course. You've had a fever," I said, but my chest tightened. I hung up, marched to my computer and searched "anemia" on the Internet.

I learned that anemia can be caused by many conditions. The bad ones, the life-threatening ones, jumped out at me. *Don't focus on those*, I told myself. Ralph's problem would be minor, easily cured with vitamins or iron tablets.

But when Dr. Whitmore called, he said the anemia wasn't related to iron deficiency and referred Ralph to a hematologist for a bone marrow aspiration. On the following Wednesday we would hear the results.

The tiny seed of anxiety inside me began to grow. Each night I woke and checked Ralph. I found him sleeping peacefully beside me, his breathing deep and regular. "*See*," I reassured myself, "*he isn't worried.*"

Ralph never worried. Nothing fazed him. Soon after we met, he invited me to see the home he'd bought in Shore Acres along Galveston Bay. When we walked into the house, we found the kitchen floor covered with two inches of water. "I must've connected the refrigerator hose wrong," Ralph said without a hint of distress. He left the room, came back with a mop and a bucket, and got to work.

Impressed by his attitude, I watched him calmly wield the mop. My former husband would have cleaned up, too, but not with such good grace. He'd have been furious that a possession of his was threatened in any way, even if it was his own fault.

"*Wow*," I thought as Ralph set things to right. "*This is the kind of man I should marry.*"

I needed someone like Ralph, because I worried constantly: about the children, money, being caught in the rain, a stain on the living room carpet, money...

Later I found more reasons to fall in love with Ralph: his easy good nature, his friendliness, and most of all his kindness and interest in my children, his willingness to include them in outings, even his patience in playing a game of Monopoly with them before we went out on New Year's Eve. He had custody of his three-year-old son Bryan and arranged his life to accommodate his child. I knew, despite our religious difference, that he was the soulmate I'd been searching for. Two years after we met, we were married.

Now, as the days moved inexorably toward Wednesday, I tried to convince myself the news from the bone marrow test would be good and afterward I'd be able to chide myself for my fears.

On Tuesday I was home for lunch when Ralph walked in. He ambled into the kitchen and began making a sandwich. "I saw the hematologist this morning," he said.

"But we're going tomorrow."

"I went today."

I swallowed and waited.

He said, "I have something called myelodysplastic syndrome."

I'd never heard of this disease but it sounded ominous. How could Ralph stand there calmly slicing tomatoes while he relayed this news? Slice, slice, as our world began slipping away.

"It's a blood cancer," he said, adding lettuce to his sandwich. They don't know much about it. I told the doctor I wanted to do a clinical trial, and he said, good, he'd refer me to the Franklin Cancer Institute in the medical center."

A cancer hospital. A place that treated a disease named for a crab. I pictured the cancer burrowing into Ralph's body, snatching organs with its pincers, squeezing the life out of them.

A wail surged inside me, but I forced it back. This wasn't about me; it was about him.

I didn't ask why he'd chosen to go to the doctor alone. I knew he'd wanted to take the blow on his own, feel it knock him backward, then pull himself up and deal with it in his own mind before he had to tell me and handle my reaction, too.

I wouldn't burden him with the response he dreaded. I went to him, hugged him and said, "You'll be okay."

"I know I will," he said. "The Cancer Institute has the best doctors."

I nodded, then pushed my unfinished lunch away and went to my computer. This time my fingers, usually so quick, fumbled on the keys. I wasn't even sure how to spell Ralph's disease. My hands chilled as I googled myelodysplastic syndrome.

Myelodysplastic syndromes: a group of diseases characterized by disruption of the production of blood cells by the bone marrow.

The website had a patients' bulletin board. I read a few postings.

"My beloved grandfather died this week of MDS."

I closed the file.

My thoughts flashed back to Yom Kippur and God's judging of our souls, deciding whether to grant life or death. A nice metaphor, I'd always thought. So, how did God decide? Did He flip a coin?

"You're getting ahead of yourself, thinking of death," I scolded. But I couldn't quiet my fears. What if Ralph were taken from me? Who would I be without him? Perhaps I would disappear. I needed his love to make me visible. I wanted to race back to the kitchen, into Ralph's arms. I wanted him to comfort me as he always did in times of trouble.

This kind of thinking was selfish. Now was my turn to be the comforter, my turn to be the strong one, even if my show of courage was a ruse.

Alone in my study with the door closed, I laid my head on my arms and shut my eyes. A few weeks ago, I'd thought about retiring from my career as a speech pathologist at the end of this school year and becoming a full-time romance writer. Ralph officed at home. I was uncertain how we'd manage being together all day every day and asked myself if I wanted that. Now I knew the answer: Yes, yes, yes.

I wanted to cry, but no tears came. My mother never cried. She said she couldn't. When my father died, she wailed and moaned, but her eyes were dry. I considered her inability to cry a failing. I didn't understand it. When I was younger, I cried over the slightest mishap: a car with a dead battery, a malfunctioning washing machine, a cancelled outing. Now my tears blocked up inside. Had I become my mother?

I don't remember what we said and did the rest of the day. I don't remember calling the children, but we must have. We were a blended family – my son and daughter and Ralph's son. We used to call ourselves the Brady Bunch.

Like the Bradys, all our offspring had different ways of coping. Bryan, Ralph's son, was laconic as usual; Michael, my son, more noticeably upset.

I don't remember what I said to Lori, my daughter, but I do recall her take-charge attitude. A veterinarian at Baylor College of Medicine, she once worked for the Cancer Institute. "I'll call the people I know there and find out who specializes in myelodysplastic syndrome," she said.

Her matter-of-fact tone calmed me. This disease could be managed. There'd be a doctor, a treatment, a cure. Yes, definitely, a cure. And so we waited for the hospital appointment, going on with our lives as usual, pretending everything was normal. Maybe it was. Maybe this little-known disease was no more than a brush with cancer. But I didn't think so.

That fall the Houston Astros battled the St. Louis Cardinals for the National League pennant. In times of stress I have always lost myself in sports. Not playing them. I was the skinny, awkward kid who was always chosen last for teams in elementary school. But watching is different. It's riveting, distracting, and you never know how the game will end. This year we both watched as the Astros put up a gallant fight but lost. They say baseball is a metaphor for life. I hoped that wasn't true.

At last the hospital called. Ralph went in for a history and more blood tests. He would have the results on October 27, in less than a week.

CHAPTER 2

October 27, 2004, was a golden afternoon, one of Houston's few crisp fall days. I hoped the mellow sunlight and the cloudless sky were an omen.

I drove to meet Ralph and Lori, who had driven together to the Gulf Coast Medical Center. I tried to focus on the pleasant weather, the children I'd seen in my speech pathology practice that morning, anything but the flutters in my stomach, the tightness in my chest.

Suddenly I remembered I'd told myself that before I left for the appointment, I would kiss the mezuzah, the small case containing a scroll from Deuteronomy that is fastened to the doors of Jewish homes. To assure them of God's protection, religious Jews place their fingertips on their lips and then on the mezuzah when they enter and leave home. I am not a particularly religious Jew, nor am I a believer in good luck charms or magic. But when I went to Austin during my father's last illness, I did not pack my black suit, reasoning that if I didn't take it, I wouldn't need it. Ralph brought my black clothing with him when he arrived for Daddy's funeral.

Now I was half way to the Medical Center and it was too late to turn back. I knew in my head that kissing the mezuzah would not affect Ralph's diagnosis or his outcome, but the worry that I neglected this promise continued to nag me.

I concentrated on how fortunate we were to live fifteen minutes from the Franklin Cancer Institute, ranked by *U.S. News and World Report* as the number one cancer hospital in the United States. People travel here from all over the world; we had only to drive down the freeway.

I pulled into Garage 2, a building I would become far too familiar with in the coming months. I found a space and walked across the street into the building that housed the physicians who held my husband's life in their hands.

Ralph and Lori were already in an examining room with pristine white walls and floors. White for beginnings, for new life. A good sign. I saw portents everywhere.

Ralph wore a long-sleeved green shirt, khaki pants and a pair of scuffed brown loafers. Pretty much what he wore every day. From his outfit one couldn't tell that today was a milestone in his life. In all our lives.

Silently, we waited. The minutes crawled by, and then the door opened and Dr. Riker, the specialist Ralph had seen last week, entered the room. A man of medium height with a receding hairline and thin lips, he wore the physician's uniform of long white coat. His trousers were precisely creased, his shoes shined to a high gloss – *a perfectionist, a no-nonsense doctor,* I told myself.

"Good afternoon, sir," he greeted my husband, then turned to me. "Madam."

I was sixty-nine years old, and no one had ever called me "madam" before.

The doctor gave Lori a perfunctory glance, then a brief nod. He listened to Ralph's heart, then sat down and leafed through the sheaf of papers centered on his desk. "Your lab tests are in," he said. "You have acute myelogenous leukemia."

Yes, no nonsense from this man. He delivered the words with the sting of a slap.

I froze, shocked into silence. I thought, *I'll remember this moment for the rest of my life.*

Ralph looked confused. "What about the myelodysplastic syndrome?"

"MDS is a precursor to leukemia. There are seven varieties of AML, the type of leukemia you have. Yours is M6, erythrocytic, in which chromosomes are transposed. It's a particularly difficult one to cure."

His words sounded like a death sentence. Doubtless Dr. Riker handed them out every day, but for us this was the one and only. I wanted to punch this doctor with his cool demeanor and disinterested tone. I felt my fists clench, hid them in my lap, and focused on my family.

Lori looked stricken, her face ashen, her lips trembling. I searched Ralph's face, trying to read his mind, his heart, but his eyes told me nothing. I had seen my husband angry, I had seen him cry, but in the face of this news his gaze on the doctor's face was steady, his hands still.

Dr. Riker handed Ralph a sheet of paper explaining his disease. Ralph read it. Swallowing hard, I leaned over to look, too.

I knew a lot about leukemia. Only a few weeks ago I had sent my editor at Silhouette Books a proposal for a romance novel in which the heroine's son had AML. Was this life imitating fiction, or had I somehow caused this disease by my choice of plots?

I glanced at Lori. Usually assertive, she, too, was stunned into silence.

I asked, "Will he have a bone marrow transplant?"

"He's too old," the doctor replied. He turned back to Ralph. "Sir, last week you mentioned wanting to participate in a clinical trial."

Ralph nodded.

"The research nurse will explain it to you." He started to get up. "You need to check into the hospital now."

"Now? Today?"

"This afternoon."

Ralph shook his head. "I can't do that. I have to make arrangements for my business." He sounded angry, his first show of emotion.

Dr. Riker grimaced, sat down again and realigned the papers. "Tomorrow, then."

"Monday."

The doctor frowned at Ralph. "Your immune system is weak; you're at risk for infection. If you get sick, we won't be able to begin treatment."

Ralph could be stubborn. His jaw clenched. "Monday."

The doctor huffed. "All right, your choice. You'll be in the protective environment – that's isolation – for a month."

A month, I thought. We'd never been separated for a more than a few days. A month was ... forever.

"You won't be allowed to leave the room or have anyone in, but each room has a window and a booth with a telephone so you can talk with visitors."

"Like prison," I remarked.

The doctor whipped around and scowled. "This hospital is not a prison," he said. "We don't keep people here if they want to leave."

Rebuked and humiliated, I stared at the floor. Had I not been staggered by the diagnosis he'd so coldly delivered, I might have snapped back at him, but I was too shaken. I would not risk any more comments.

Dr. Riker picked up the chart. "Well, sir, the research nurse will explain everything about the clinical trial."

Suddenly Lori said, "And if he decides to have the standard treatment, then what do we do?"

The doctor glared at her as if she were a fifth-grade student speaking out of turn in class. He addressed Ralph. "Leave," he replied. "Go back to your regular doctor. Standard treatment is not what the Cancer Institute is about."

While the three of us stared at him in shock, he continued. "Where would medical science be," he asked, "if we just gave standard treatments? Fifty years behind where we are now."

Had there been a soapbox in the room, he surely would have jumped up on it. His voice rose. "This is the largest leukemia center in the world. Clinical trials are *what we do.*"

"I said I was interested in a clinical trial," Ralph said quietly.

"Good. I'll send in the nurse." Without a word of farewell, Dr. Riker left the room.

Within moments, we heard a knock and the nurse entered. A light-skinned African-American, she was a heavy-set woman who nodded to us pleasantly. Or perhaps she wasn't pleasant. I don't recall. Even a glare would have seemed warmer than Dr. Riker's icy delivery.

"All nine other patients on this protocol are in remission," she told us. At last, some good news.

She explained the treatment procedure and recited the litany of possible side effects – rash, nausea, hair loss, gastrointestinal problems, vision problems, fatigue; the list went on and on. She discussed the protective environment. No plants in the room, no fresh fruits or vegetables.

"Can I bring my laptop with me?" Ralph asked. He was a computer consultant; the laptop was his most treasured possession.

"Yes," she said, and I heard his deep sigh of relief.

He glanced over the consent form and scribbled his name,

got instructions for checking into the hospital, and still numb with shock from the diagnosis and Dr. Riker's tongue lashing, we left.

Lori went back to work. Hand in hand, Ralph and I walked outside into the sunlight, which no longer looked bright.

We were silent as we began the drive home through afternoon traffic. Dozens of questions tumbled around in my mind. I felt as if I were on a tiny raft, tossed into a lonely sea. Ralph would be in the hospital a month. Who would I lean on?

Thoughts crowded my mind. Where was Ralph's insurance policy? The extra set of car keys? The key to the safe deposit box? How would we take care of medical bills?

I wondered what Ralph was thinking. How to break the news to his family in Iowa? How to tell his clients? Who would take care of their technology problems for the month he was hospitalized?

"We have to make a list," I said.

"No."

"But ..."

"No."

His illness, his choice. I didn't protest, but I felt a window close between us. I could see him on the other side, but I couldn't reach him. Would this be our future?

CHAPTER 3

During the next few days Ralph said little. Had I been the one facing cancer, I would have spilled all my fears into his willing ears. But that was not his way. Only once that weekend did I get a glimpse of his inner turmoil. He'd spoken with all his clients about his situation. "I told them Mark and David (his employees) would take care of them and I'd be in contact while I was in the hospital. They all said that was fine and asked me to keep them informed about my progress and said they wished me well." He looked down at his hands. "I was afraid they'd find someone else to do their computer work."

I reached for his hand and squeezed. So many times his big hand had encircled mine, giving me support and strength – when my father died, when my son Michael had a heart attack and bypass surgery at age thirty-four. But Ralph couldn't comfort me now and, much as I longed to, I couldn't ask it of him; this was my time to be the strong one.

Wherever I looked were signs of how different our lives had suddenly become. In our driveway stood an RV. Fully loaded, with king size bed, microwave, and TV, its width spanned the driveway.

When we were in Iowa the summer before, crossing the state to spend a day with Ralph's brother, we picked up a flyer describing points of interest. "I have an idea. Let's travel across the country, coast to coast," I suggested.

To my surprise, Ralph agreed. We spent the rest of the drive planning our imaginary trip. "Next summer," I said.

"Later. Maybe the summer after."

"Later," was Ralph's favorite word; "just a minute" his favorite phrase. So I was astonished when a month afterward I returned from a trip with my sister to find the RV parked in our drive. "Surprise!" he said. We decided to take a trial trip to the Texas Hill Country in October.

Now October was almost over and the RV sat by the house,

an ungainly monster, the symbol of a trip I somehow knew we would never take.

While Ralph made arrangements for his business, I attended a Saturday workshop on language disabilities at the University of Houston. As the morning session got under way, I saw colleagues I'd known for years, their expressions absorbed, their pencils busy. I resented them all. They would return to their homes when the lecture concluded, go out to dinner or a movie with husbands or lovers, laugh together, complain about the traffic, make love. And the beauty, the miracle of such ordinary things would not cross their minds. Their day-to-day lives would continue, unquestioned, unappreciated. Ours wouldn't.

Usually a meticulous note taker, that morning I could barely concentrate. Only one comment from the lecture imprinted itself on my mind, to resurface time and time again over the next months. Near tears, the speaker, a renowned authority in language-learning disabilities, told us about the recent birth of her grandson. The delivery was difficult and the infant suffered a birth injury. With her expertise, she knew what the future might hold for this child. "On the way home from the hospital," she said, "I totaled my car." I feared that during this time of crisis, I would do the same.

Sunday, before he entered the hospital, Ralph stayed awake all night, working on his computer. I don't know what he was typing – instructions about his customers, probably – but he couldn't, or wouldn't, stop. Every hour I woke and trudged into the room he used as a home office. "What are you doing? Please come to bed."

"I have work to do." A mountain of papers spilled across his desk; open folders lay on the floor beside a half-packed black leather bag. His fingers rushed across the keyboard.

"Please."

"I'll be there in a minute."

Finally, near morning he came to bed. He shucked off his clothes, lay down naked beside me and pulled me close. I wanted us to be together, skin to skin; I struggled out of my nightgown, lay flush against him and hugged him. He was warm, solid, but his muscles were wire-tight.

Would he survive the treatment? If he did, would he be a different person when he came home?

We didn't talk, we didn't make love; we just held one another close until morning came and the first day of our cancer journey began. At 7:00 a.m. we walked into the Franklin Cancer Institute. One of many buildings in the busy Gulf Coast Medical Center, it was an immense pink granite structure. A grand piano, dwarfed by the size of the room, stood near the front door. Later I would see patients and their families grouped around it while volunteers performed. The music – show tunes, old favorites, classical pieces – provided an escape from cancer. Chairs and couches were grouped around the sides of the room, and at the back was a case filled with porcelain birds. The center of the huge lobby was topped by skylights three stories high. I felt we had entered a cathedral, a temple of healing.

Gazing up, I somehow expected to see a symbolic beam of sunshine. Instead the morning was dim, with ominous, low-hanging clouds.

I focused on the room's side walls, with pictures and stories of people who had beaten cancer, as Ralph wheeled his suitcase across the lobby. In it were his robe and slippers, socks, underwear, magazines and the morning edition of the Houston *Chronicle*. Under his other arm was his ever-present computer. Never willing to part with it, he brought it along on every trip we took. I often felt we were a *menage a trois*: Ralph, the laptop, and me.

From the moment we entered the hospital I became a leukemia wife. In the next year I would expand my vocabulary to include words like afaresis, Tacrolimus, allogeneic, neutropenic, creatinin. Acronyms would roll off my tongue: AML, CVC, BMT, and the sinister GVHD (graft versus host disease). In twelve months I would visit Ralph in eleven hospital rooms on four different floors, meet with thirty specialists, spend over $1500 on parking, lose my car twice in the garage, lose my temper with nurses, doctors, two social workers and the patient advocate, and watch 137 reruns of "Law and Order."

That first morning after hugging Ralph, I left the hospital and drove to work. I was almost an hour early, and I decided I would go to Starbucks, even though I'd eaten breakfast at home. When I'm tense, I crave sweets, and I desperately wanted a cranberry muffin. I could already taste the tart berries and smell coffee roasting. But as I drove away from the Medical Center, the clouds opened and rain gushed forth, pounding the roof and hood of my car. I turned on the windshield wipers and tightened my grasp on the wheel. *Forget Starbucks*, I thought, and drove straight to work.

When I went back to the hospital at noon, there were no parking spaces. Because of the rain, every garage in walking distance of the cancer hospital was full. I gave my keys to the valet in front of the hospital and went in to find Ralph in a cubicle in the Ambulatory Care Department, chatting amiably with a nurse who was placing a central venous catheter, a soft plastic tube through which he would receive IV fluids and chemotherapy drugs, in his chest. "Most people can't tolerate this procedure," she said. "Your husband is a great patient."

Ralph gave me a smug smile. It reminded me of our cruise to Antarctica several years earlier, when he strolled along the deck without a parka, with the same self-satisfied grin. No sissy-boy stuff for Ralph.

I'm a sissy. Seeing the site where my husband's body was cut, I felt sick to my stomach. Cancer wasn't a crab; it was a shark. It would eat him up, piece by piece. I turned away so he wouldn't read the horror in my eyes.

That evening I went back for a longer visit. I didn't want to go home. I feared I'd be unable to sleep. Ralph rarely traveled because his clients for his computer consulting company were in the Houston area. I wasn't used to being alone at night, and I was as scared as I'd been when I was a little girl and imagined monsters invading my room in the dark.

I was half way home when the blinding rain began again. My fears turned from being alone to getting home at all. By the time I arrived, the rain had slowed. I went inside and fell into bed, exhausted.

When I woke, the clock beside me read 6:30. I sat up and glanced around. Toby, my black and white cat, greeted me with a meow. I hadn't wakened once, hadn't had a nightmare. I'd made it through that first night. Never again would I be afraid of being alone.

CHAPTER 4

Tuesday, November 2, 2004: Election Day. On my way to work I drove past Kolter Elementary School where we voted. I pondered the presidential choices: Bush or Kerry? Even on Election Day, I had no strong preference.

Ralph had prudently voted absentee. No use asking him which candidate he preferred. A Midwesterner and staunch conservative, he'd never voted for a Democrat and never intended to. Often our votes canceled each other out, but over the years he'd managed to steer me from ultra-liberal to semi-moderate.

One long ago primary election I was at the polls, giving out leaflets for a state senatorial candidate, when Ralph parked across the street and strode toward the school. He'd been working in the yard. His shirt was damp, his face streaked with perspiration and his hair disheveled. "Here comes a Democrat," the woman beside me predicted.

"Oh, no, he's a Republican," I said.

"No way."

"I know he is," I told her. "He's my husband."

This election morning, I decided I would vote at noon, and no matter which candidate I chose, I would cheer Ralph by telling him I voted the straight Republican ticket. Not that he'd believe me, but at least he'd laugh.

But at 10:30 he called. "Can you come for lunch? I'm going into isolation at 2:00."

I met him is the family room outside the isolation wing. He handed me the phone. "You can call in your lunch order," he said.

Fancy, I thought. I dialed the number he gave me.

"Room Service."

Like a hotel. I ordered a chicken salad sandwich. Fifteen minutes later my lunch arrived, presented by a tuxedo-clad waiter. Was this a strategy to make cancer patients feel they were staying in a world class resort?

Tuxedos or not, majestic lobby notwithstanding, this floor

still looked and smelled like a hospital.

After lunch we went to Ralph's room. The time had come for him to tell his mother he had leukemia. He'd arranged for his sister to be with her when he called. His voice shook when he told her. Tears welled in his eyes.

He'd shed no tears when he told me his diagnosis. Perhaps it was harder for him to contain his emotions with his mother; perhaps he felt he had to appear stronger for me. Or maybe because his mother couldn't see him, he thought she wouldn't notice the tremor in his voice. He quickly regained control of himself and assured her he was in the world's best cancer hospital and he'd be fine. I knew his mom responded that she'd be praying for him. What he didn't tell her or anyone else in his evangelical Christian family was that when he entered the hospital, he'd listed himself as Jewish.

A nurse stepped into the room. "Mr. Zirkelbach, we're ready to move you to isolation."

Ralph's face paled as he nodded to the nurse. He reached for my hand and held it so tight my fingers hurt. He pulled me close and kissed me. We would not touch again for a month.

I left the hospital, drove slowly to my office and spent the afternoon immersed in therapy sessions. I learned early to compartmentalize my life. My college boyfriend was diagnosed with thyroid cancer. Soon after that I began my practicum in speech pathology in the public schools. I was devastated, but each day, the moment I entered the school, I put everything else out of my mind. Now, I promised myself, I would do the same.

I arrived at my office in time to check my voice mail and return a few phone calls before my first afternoon appointment, a lively four-year-old with a language disorder. My calls done, I shut my eyes for a moment of relaxation. Deep breath ...

What was Ralph doing, locked away in his isolation room? Would the chemo make him sick? Was he ...

The waiting room bell rang. I shut my thoughts away and opened the door. "Hi, Brett."

Chocolate-brown eyes sparkled. "What we gonna do today?"

"Say, 'Hi, Miss Thelma.' Then you can ask me."

"Hi, Miss Thelma." He followed me into my therapy room.

"What we do?"

"What *are* we *going* to do? We're going to make a picture with stick-on people." I took a box of materials from the bookcase filled with picture books, puzzles, and elementary school readers and bypassed the child-size table that Ralph had refinished. "This will be fun. Let's sit on the floor ... right here."

We settled in the corner beneath a bulletin board decorated with a kitten calendar and a picture drawn by a child I worked with. I opened my box and took out the background scene of a town and a sheet of stickers. "Here we go. What shall we put on the picture first?"

"That one." Brett gestured to a boy on a bike.

"No pointing. Use words."

"The boy."

"Look, there are so many boys. Which one?"

"The boy with hair ... brown hair," he said.

My career as a speech pathologist spanned thirty years. I didn't have to think about what to do. Automatically, I elicited more information about each choice Brandon made.

Near the end of our session Brett said, "The trucks now?"

"Are we going to play with the trucks? Yes." This was his reward for working hard.

"The fire truck's breaked. The wheel comed off," he observed. "Let's get Miss Karlene. She fix it."

It hadn't taken Brett many sessions to determine that "Miss Thelma" was mechanically challenged and that my partner Karlene was the fix-it lady in the office. Of course, at home that was Ralph's job. Karlene quickly reassembled the truck. Brett and I finished our session, and the next child arrived.

By 6:00 I was worn out from thoughts of Ralph that inched their way into my forced peppiness and from the stress of shutting my worries away.

Derek, my last client, was a kindergartner, the second child I'd worked with in his family. His articulation had improved notably, and at the end of his session I told him, "We'll start a new sound next time. It'll be your last one and then you'll graduate."

"Wow, I'm doing gweat."

"Yeah, you are."

With a handful of goldfish crackers for a treat, he dashed into the waiting room to tell his mom the good news.

On Thursday we would begin the dreaded /r/, the bane of every speech pathologist's existence because it's such a difficult sound to demonstrate and often takes a long time to master. A mother once told me her daughter complained the sound was too hard. "Who cares about wabbits and wobots anyway?" she grumbled.

I flipped through my articulation cards and selected /r/ pictures for our next meeting. R for raincoat, R for rooster. I gathered my purse and briefcase. R for Ralph.

I left my office at 6:45. Ten minutes later I passed our precinct polls. I could easily have rushed in and voted, but I was too tired. I drove to the Medical Center.

At the entrance to the hospital's isolation floor was a sign instructing visitors to cover their shoes with paper booties from a box nearby and to clean their hands with antiseptic. Since my feet are small, the large blue booties slipped on easily over my shoes. I felt like a clown as I awkwardly shuffled through the heavy door and down the hall to Ralph's room.

I opened the door to the visitors' space. It was no bigger than a closet and almost as dark. A window looked into Ralph's room, and a telephone for communicating with him sat on a small table. They'd tried to disguise the visitors' room with chairs upholstered in a flowery fabric, but I wasn't fooled. No matter what Dr. Riker said, this place was a prison.

Ralph's room looked like any other hospital room except for a free-standing toilet. To protect from germs, isolation rooms did not have plumbing. I had been told the reason for this caution, but I felt the lack of privacy robbed patients of their dignity, reduced them to animals whose bodily functions were performed in public.

How had this calamity happened? Only a month ago we were two ordinary people, living ordinary lives: a little bored really, a little anxious about what old age held for us. We were healthy then, but didn't rejoice over that gift.

When I was young and upset about something, my mother would annoy me by saying, "At least you have your health." Tell that to a sixteen-year-old who wasn't invited to the spring dance. To a cancer patient's wife, the words suddenly made sense.

Wearily, I sat down in the claustrophobic space and picked up the telephone.

The first thing Ralph said to me that Tuesday evening was, "You'd better buy me some pajamas. These hospital gowns are crap." The next thing was, "Did you vote?"

That question was "so Ralph." "No."

He frowned toward the glass. "You should have."

"Think of it this way," I answered. The 'other' candidate got one less vote."

"True," he agreed.

Through the window, I watched TV with Ralph as Bush won the election and my Republican husband grinned triumphantly.

◆ ◆ ◆

In the hospital Ralph was patient number 630967, but he did everything possible to be seen as an individual. By the end of the week, he had made himself thoroughly at home. A friend brought a printer, a copy machine, and six file boxes, which were now lined up in his room. "Good Lord," Lori said when she visited, "this looks just like his office at home."

The nurses enjoyed Ralph's upbeat attitude and remarked upon his endurance of the chemo and his ability to keep working.

He talked about technology to the nurses and anyone else who would listen; computers were his passion. When he graduated from college at Iowa State, he took a job with Celanese Chemical where he worked on their huge mainframe computer. He loved to recount his midwinter trip to Kingsville, Texas for his interview. He wasn't sure whether to accept the position Celanese offered, but when he returned from sunny Texas to O'Hare Airport in Chicago and found his automobile engine frozen, he made his decision.

Later when he opened his own business, he called it Solution Providers. He considered himself a problem solver and welcomed the challenge of setting up computer networks and overcoming glitches. He got to know his clients and their families, even their pets, and enjoyed his interaction with them.

He did the same with the nurses; he chatted with them and learned their backgrounds. He was especially drawn to a young nurse from India who was looking forward to a vacation home in a few weeks. He questioned her about her country, her culture, and what had brought her to America.

He also liked to brag to the nurses about his wife, the romance writer. I had a book coming out in February called *Stranger in Her Arms*, and he posted a picture of the cover on the wall in his room.

For my part, I operated under the adage, "Live one day at a time." I'd never thought this was realistic, but I noticed I was actually doing this. Each day I read the printout from the lab, listing all of Ralph's counts. Each time I read them I was relieved we'd gotten through one more day.

I'm a counter. Five years is the benchmark in cancer. Five years, 1825 days. Seventeen days since his diagnosis. 1808 left to go.

Of course, I worried about the problems of daily life. What would I do if my car broke down? Should we install an alarm system in the house? Should we put our house up for sale and move to a smaller, less costly space? A new apartment building had recently opened near us and I passed it on the way to work. I began to think of it as a fallback.

Nevertheless, since Ralph's treatment seemed to be going well, I tried to make my days as normal as possible. Most evenings I visited Ralph at the hospital, but on Thursdays my friend Marla and I resumed our weekly book discussions. Feeling it was an obligation, a rite of passage, we were reading *Ulysses*. We hated it. Eventually we gave up, leaving Leopold Bloom in the midst of his lunch. I went out to lunch with friends, attended board meetings of the University of Houston Communication Disorders Alumni Association. I wrote reports, paid bills, visited my mother at her nursing home.

At the hospital I attended a support group on the isolation floor. Like all families linked by illness, the group members bonded quickly. We may not have known one anothers' full names, but we knew our loved ones' histories, diagnoses, and current status. We shared news about our patient's white cell count, nausea, bowel obstructions, rashes. You might say we learned about each others' family members from the inside out. And I admit to being secretly elated when Ralph's platelet count climbed faster than another patient's or he made any other sign of rapid progress.

Bolstered by his progress and still waiting to hear about my latest proposal to Silhouette Books, I decided to write a book about Ralph's illness. I would call it *Leukemia Wife*, and it would be a cheerful, upbeat account of his diagnosis and cure, a how-to book for spouses of cancer patients. I began keeping notes on our daily experiences.

I thought I was doing well in supporting Ralph and keeping my own spirits high. And then I ran into a youngster I had worked with several years earlier. "Hi, Allan," I said. "How are you?"

"Fine," he answered, surveying me through narrowed eyes. "I haven't seen you in a while. How old are you now, about a hundred?"

Stress ages you, but a hundred? Back in my therapy room I reached for my mirror and then put it away. Better not to look.

♦♦♦

One day in the third week of his treatment, I arrived at the hospital, where Ralph greeted me with a scowl. "People from the bone marrow transplant department came to see me."

"But the doctor said you weren't a candidate for a transplant."

"That's what I thought, and I didn't like the hard sell. They were like damn telemarketers, trying to push me into something I don't even know if I need."

A sales pitch? *No*, I thought. *It must be a message that chemo is useless. They expect the treatment to fail.*

"If I have a transplant," Ralph continued, "I'll have to come to the hospital every day for a year."

I hadn't cried when I learned Ralph was ill, but that evening while I drove home, my tears flowed uncontrollably. Sobbing, I called Lori.

One of her colleagues had a son who had leukemia. "The most important thing to know about a transplant is once he starts the process, he can't go back," she said. "After they kill off Ralph's bone marrow, if the transplant doesn't engraft, he'll have nothing to fall back on."

Now I was truly terrified. I resolved not to let Ralph know. I would keep this new fear locked up inside with the others. Better for him to be angry than scared.

The next day Lori called the hospital's bone marrow department, and one of the nursing staff agreed to see us after hours to explain the transplant process.

Lori, Michael and I met her on Thursday evening. The clinic was deserted and eerily quiet. The nurse invited us into an office and quickly explained the procedure. They used stem cells, not bone marrow. The best match would be a sibling. Ralph had four. Each had a twenty-five per cent chance of matching. She suggested we begin the screening process immediately because it took a long time.

Then she began to list complications of stem cell transplant.

"Intestinal disorders." Uncomfortable, but I guessed he could live with that.

"Vision problems." Could he drive? Read? Or did she mean he would be blind?

"Jaundice." Ugly, but what else did it imply? Then I remembered. Liver disease. You had only one liver so that meant ...

"Graft versus host disease. The donor cells reject the patient's own cells. It can happen any time after transplant. It may last for years."

Was the cure worse than the disease?

I wondered if I sounded this disinterested when I gave parents their kids' diagnoses. "Your child has dyslexia. It affects not just reading words but comprehension, spelling, writing, everything in school." Did they feel as stunned as I did now? Did they want to throw something at me? I wanted to shout at this calm, composed woman, "How would you feel listening to this if the patient were your husband?"

But of course, he wasn't her husband, and she was only doing her job.

I remembered that a few days before he entered the hospital, Ralph asked me, "How long do you think I'll live if I don't have chemo?"

Dr. Riker had said he was at risk for infection without immediate hospitalization, so I assumed the time would be short. I blurted out the first answer that came to mind. "A week, I guess."

If I'd read on the Internet about average life expectancy with AML, I hadn't absorbed it. Apparently neither had Ralph. I think people in crisis tend to take in only as much as they can manage.

Today I ask myself if he hadn't had treatment and all it entailed, how long would he have had? Without treatment, would his last days have been peaceful? Did my off-the-cuff answer of a week push him in an unwanted direction?

That evening I vowed that whatever choice he made would be his alone. I would not influence his decision about the transplant. However I felt, I would be silent.

CHAPTER 5

While I pondered stem cell transplants and took classes on how to care for Ralph's central catheter, my mother was dying.

Three months earlier she'd turned one hundred. For the past sixteen years she'd lived in a nursing home a few miles from our house. Most of that time she was frail, both in body and mind. Dementia robbed her of her memories. She was alive, yet not alive.

Now she suffered from congestive heart failure and frequent infections. For over a year, she'd been incontinent, unable to walk without assistance, and uncommunicative. The only time she'd spoken to me in the last twelve months was when I accidentally tripped and lunged against her bed. "What the hell are you doing?" she shouted, startling me, sounding nothing like herself, a woman who rarely raised her voice.

In September my sister and I agreed to put her on hospice. I sobbed as I read the book they gave me about dying. As time went on, I could see end-of-life signs clearly. She refused food, her breathing was shallow, she "picked" at herself. But I was so involved in Ralph's illness I had few emotional resources left for my mother.

On November 22 the hospice nurse called me. "Your mother's blood pressure is very low."

I called Ralph and asked him to phone my sister Betty in Miami and gave him a list of others to call later. Then I hurried to the nursing home.

Mother lay in bed, her eyes closed, her breathing shallow. She was a tiny woman, barely five feet and less than ninety pounds, but now she seemed so small she barely took up any space in the narrow bed.

I reached for her gnarled hand. Her fingernails still had remnants of red polish: Revlon Fire and Ice.

Sixteen years ago when she came to the nursing home, her mind was still alert enough to take in the change in her surroundings. She detested the home, hated being around "all those old people." One morning when I took her for a ride, she patted the passenger seat and said with a smirk, "Twenty-five years, and *you'll* be sitting here."

Time passed and her confusion mounted. One day she asked, "Did I have a husband? Did I die before him?"

And now her death was near.

The rabbi came in and said a prayer and offered to call the funeral home and our synagogue in Austin. Caroline Waters, Mother's long-time sitter, and I kept a vigil by her bed.

When Caroline left, I moved closer, laid my head on the bed and put my hand on Mother's arm. I'd shed many tears for her, living in her shadow world, not knowing who I was or even who she was. Now, leaning against her, patting her soft, fragile skin, I told her how much I'd loved her reading to me as a child, listening to all my problems, caring for me, being my mother.

Suddenly, her eyes flew open, she gave a little gasp and her mouth snapped shut. It seemed as if she took a last clear look at life. Then in seconds, her mouth fell slack, her eyes closed, and she stopped breathing.

I called my sister. "She's gone."

There was silence on the line. I think Betty believed this would never happen. Finally, she said, "Ronnie and I have our plane reservations. We'll be there tomorrow afternoon."

Jewish tradition requires funerals be as soon after death as possible. Had she been buried in Houston, the ceremony would have been Tuesday but our family plot was in Austin. We decided the funeral would be Wednesday afternoon. That would give Betty's children time to fly in from Atlanta and Chicago.

By the time I got home, the cantor from Mother's congregation in Austin was on the phone. His deep, soothing voice calmed me. I told him our wishes and thanked him for calling.

I never dreamed I would be making funeral arrangements by myself. I always had Ralph to fall back on. Now when I needed him most, he was out of reach. He felt helpless, too, unable to do anything but make a few phone calls. My friend told me when he called about my mother, he cried because he couldn't do more to help me.

I was certain I didn't know what to do about the funeral, but by the end of the day I realized I was managing. Bolstered by loving phone calls from Ralph and family members, I took care of everything ... or I thought I did.

The next morning my confidence was shattered. Just to be sure we all agreed on the time of the funeral, I called the cantor. "I haven't been able to find anyone to perform the service for you," he said.

And why hadn't he called to mention this, I wondered, but said nothing.

He continued. "If you can have the funeral in the morning, I'll do it, but my family and I are leaving town at noon."

"We can't. My sister's children won't get in until 1:00."

"I've called five rabbis," the cantor continued, "and no one is available."

"No one?" I managed.

"It's the holidays."

Yes, Wednesday was the day before Thanksgiving. But I had enough to deal with: a dead mother, a possibly dying husband, my own quicksilver temper. "I thought rabbis were like doctors," I said, getting teary. "I thought they were on call."

"It's the holidays," he repeated.

"My family were members of the Austin congregation for sixty years," I said, my voice rising. "They donated the Eternal Light to the synagogue. They donated a Torah. How do you think my mother would feel to know that no one could find the time to say a prayer at her grave?"

"It's ... "

"You don't have to tell me. It's the holidays. Shall we just leave her at the funeral home here until Thanksgiving is over? Oh, no, I forgot. Next week is Chanukah. That's a holiday, too."

By now the calm, kind cantor had lost patience, too. "I'll see what I can do," he said.

He called me back an hour later to say he'd found a rabbi from a new, small congregation who would perform the service. After I hung up, I curled up on the bed and cried. From embarrassment at my temper tantrum, from anger, from grief. Then I got up and got busy finalizing our plans.

◆◆◆

In Austin on Wednesday my sister, her husband and I met briefly with Rabbi Chaim Bernstein, and then went to our lawyer's office to go over Mother's will. She had left a bequest to the synagogue.

Betty and I looked at each other. Later we agreed we'd both had the same thought: no way would our mother want a synagogue that wouldn't perform her burial service to have a cent of her money. Until dementia erased her memory, she had the recall of an elephant. Especially for hurts, upsets, embarrassments. For years she reminded me of the time I yelled at Betty when I taught her to ride a two-wheel bike or the day I didn't come in when called and she thought I'd been kidnapped and became so upset she developed a migraine.

Lucky for the synagogue, she'd never have to remember their slight. But we did, and we never donated that money.

After leaving the attorney's office, we ate lunch and drove to the cemetery, passing Summit View, the street where we grew up. I craned my neck to catch a glimpse of our old house, a multi-colored Tudor style brick with an L-shaped red concrete porch at the front and side. That house held so many memories. No matter where I've lived, the house on Summit View has always been Home.

My clearest memories of home are smells: the clean, sharp odor of the cedar closet, chicken roasting in the oven, the citrus fragrance of magnolia in May and the sweet, romantic scent of jasmine in July; newly mown grass on summer afternoons when the yard man came, gutted candle wax on Friday nights after the Sabbath candles burned down. When my sister was small, I thought her skin smelled like cucumbers. Daddy smelled of cigarettes, Mother carried the faint tinge of face powder.

Our house faded into the distance. Now others lived there and smelled the magnolias in spring, and Mother, our last link to home, was gone.

Long ago, Mother read to me. Fairy tales, *Heidi, Bambi*. One summer when I had an eye operation, she must have read twenty *Bobbsey Twins* books.

She hated cooking but loved to bake. Whenever she made a pie, she let me make a miniature one for Daddy in my toy baking pan. Mmm, the smell of cherry pie baking. And the taste of it, warm and tart and topped with chocolate ice cream.

When I was small, Mother and I took walks together. One of my favorites was down a steep hill called Rainbow Bend. The name made the street seem magical. One of the houses near the foot of the hill had a fish pond, and we always stopped to look at it, to admire the garden and the large, lazy goldfish.

Although she wasn't social and didn't have many friends of her own, Mother always welcomed my sister's and my friends. A few years ago, I received a letter from a long-ago schoolmate, recalling a birthday party at our house. My classmate came from a large family without much money and had never seen an electric refrigerator. She mentioned standing in our kitchen, staring at it, and how kind my mother had been, offering her juice from a pitcher, an undreamed of luxury for the little girl. I cherish that letter and the thought that Mother made such a lasting impression.

At the cemetery we drove through the gate and along the winding road to the Jewish section. A tent was set up; the grave yawned before it.

Before the coffin was closed, we took a last look at Mother, In keeping with Jewish tradition she lay in a wooden casket, wrapped in a white shroud. She'd always looked young for her age; in death she looked far older than her hundred years. She was small and shrunken, her skin sallow.

She'd spent a long time dying, her brain and body ebbing away. Now she would be at peace beside my father.

The afternoon was cold and windy. I huddled in my jacket and listened as Rabbi Bernstein said the Kaddish prayer, my lips moving as he spoke.

My sister read a piece I had written about Mother that had been published in the Houston *Chronicle* on Mother's Day several years earlier:

I lost my mother eight years ago.
The woman who lives in a nursing home
a few miles from my house is not the mother I knew...

We said the Kaddish, the mourners' prayer. The rabbi pinned a torn black ribbon on each family member's lapel to symbolize the tear in the family circle, the casket was lowered, and each mourner poured a spadeful of earth onto it.

Mother now lay beneath the dry winter grass, this woman who often told my sister and me, "I know you better than you know yourselves."

No one would ever know us that well again.

◆◆◆

The next day Betty, Ronnie and I drove back to Houston, stopping for our Thanksgiving meal at Steak and Ale. While Ronnie and I waited in the car, Betty went inside to inquire about seating. She came out chuckling. "They told me all their tables were booked and I said, 'Oh, you lost our reservation,' so they said they'd find us a spot."

Betty's "white lie" made me laugh too, something I sorely needed on this holiday which was so special to our family. Every Thanksgiving I cooked sweet potatoes, cranberry sauce, spinach casserole, strawberry jello salad and a dessert that varied from year to year. Ralph was in charge of the turkey and dressing. He always prepared two kinds of dressing, plain for those of us with "normal" taste buds and jalapeno dressing, Ralph's own creation, for those who craved spice. Each year our holiday ritual included, "Ralph, this is the best turkey and the best dressing you've ever made."

Now, with Ralph locked away in his isolation room and my mother gone, I yearned for our usual family dinner. Still I was glad for my sister and brother-in-law's company and our recollections of Mother.

When we got home, Caroline, Mother's sitter, called to say she'd cleaned out Mother's room. She brought the clothes over, and Betty and I picked out a few things we wanted. I chose two sweatsuits I had given Mother for recent occasions – we wore the same size – and a Gucci handbag she had for years. We gave the rest to Caroline, who said through tears, "I feel like my own mother died."

After we hugged Caroline and she drove away, we went to the Cancer Institute. Betty said she was relieved to see that, except for a rash from the chemo, Ralph was still himself.

CHAPTER 6

The following Tuesday as I waddled down the hall in my oversize booties to the visitors' closet, the nurse stopped me. "You can go into his room."

"But ..."

"He's being discharged tomorrow. No more isolation."

I pushed open the door. Ralph met me with a huge grin. "I wanted to surprise you," he said. "I'm getting out a day early."

I couldn't think of anything to say. I just sat, mirroring his smile. Freed from "prison." Home. Back to life.

The next day, in preparation for his release, I had to pass the test on caring for his central veinous catheter. Visual motor activities are not my forte. I took the catheter instruction class twice and read the booklet the instructor gave out, but I knew I couldn't pass the test. Just a glimpse of the catheter, an alien thing implanted in Ralph's flesh, made me squeamish.

The tech who was to observe me arrived and took a seat by Ralph's bed. "Let's get started."

I began fumbling immediately. "Can I use the instruction book?"

"No."

Why not? I wondered. I'd be referring to it at home.

"Go ahead," she ordered. I tried awkwardly to put on the glove and set out the materials. The lady pursed her lips. "Didn't you read the book?"

"Yes, last week."

Her lips tightened even more. "You should have read it *this* week."

At that point my temper kicked in. "I'm sorry," I said nastily. "I was busy burying my mother."

Before the woman could respond with anything more than a gasp, Ralph intervened. "I'll be here at the hospital every day for blood work. Can't a nurse change the dressings and give my wife time to pass the test?"

The woman huffed and nodded, packed up her equipment and stomped out of the room.

I glared after her. "Maybe when I pass it, she'll give me a little prize, like I give the kids I work with."

"I don't think so," Ralph replied with a chuckle.

Eventually I did pass the test. But usually Ralph had his dressing changed at the hospital. At home, he talked me through the procedure. Once he asked a nurse at the hospital to redo a job I had performed the night before. "My wife had a headache," he lied. "Her hands were shaky."

♦♦♦

By the time Ralph was actually released from the hospital, it was evening. On the way home we stopped at the drug store and then the grocery. Ralph was delighted to be out in the world again. He put on his duck-bill mask and wandered the aisles of the supermarket, gazing at the displays. He bought yogurt, he chose soup and bread and tea. Afterward, he settled in the car as if he'd spent the best evening of his life. And then we were home at last.

Of course, there were restrictions. He had to wear a mask when he went out; he was not to go into crowded places. Although he was in remission, he was not allowed to drive until his platelet count reached 40. He could play with our two cats but had to wash his hands afterward, and they could not sleep on our bed. He could not eat fresh fruits or vegetables.

There could be no plants in the house and no gardening. "Aha," I said. "Now I can kill the Monster."

The Monster was a split-leaf philodendron that lived on our patio. Although I can't remember, I suppose it was once a small plant, but over the years it grew until it spread from one side of the patio to the other. Its roots had made a hole in the wooden planks. Its leaves were enormous. It was our own – or Ralph's own – plant from "The Little Shop of Horrors."

Since his illness, Ralph's emotions had become fragile. His eyes teared. "Don't," he said. "Promise me you won't kill it."

Darn, I thought. "All right."

Over time the plant has inched closer to the wall of the house. Some dark night I'm sure it will push through the glass of my bedroom window and strangle me in my sleep. But I made a promise and I've kept it. The Monster will remain unmolested on my patio as long as it and I live.

♦♦♦

As the month of December passed, we pretended life was normal. I continued making notes for my intended book on how to be a cancer survivor's wife. Ralph kept as busy as he was before his illness.

I felt the absence of my mother. Her self and her spirit had died long ago, but the silent hollow-eyed woman in the nursing home still connected me to the person she used to be. Every time I drove by the nursing home, I automatically started to turn in that direction.

Although I missed her, I remembered well that Mother was not all sweetness and light. She wasn't above cattiness.

She did not like Ralph. Reason number one: He wasn't Jewish. Although she never explicitly expressed her opposition – after all, I was a divorced woman in my thirties when Ralph and I married – she frequently made snide remarks in his presence. These appeared to be comments made without forethought, but I could tell by the sly expression in her eyes and the tightening of her lips that they were deliberate barbs. Ralph handled her veiled taunts with grace, usually ignoring them.

Often when we were in Austin, he avoided Mother by leaving the house. He did this because he knew she didn't like him, and she disliked him even more because he did this. She was suspicious of his disappearances. Although I knew he simply drove around, browsing in stores or visiting spots of interest because he showed me the photos he'd taken, Mother was certain there was some nefarious purpose in his absences. She never said this aloud, but she glared at Ralph when he returned. He ignored her frowns, which annoyed her even more.

While I mourned the complicated woman who was my mother, Ralph made daily trips to the hospital. Through a business associate, he found a driver, a man named Keith, who was as liberal as Ralph was conservative. The following summer Keith would travel to Crawford, Texas to meet Cindy Sheehan, the war protester, and to voice his own opposition to the Iraq war in front of the Bush ranch. Meanwhile, he and Ralph enjoyed political sparring. Usually no one could out-

argue Ralph on politics, but Keith came close, and I rejoiced that
he kept Ralph alert and involved in the world around him.

Christmas carols resounded at the grocery store. Of course,
being Jewish, I don't celebrate Christmas, but I grew up
when carols and Christmas pageants were part of the school
curriculum. I knew the songs and usually enjoyed them and
embraced the joy of the holiday season. Not this year. Every
time I heard a Christmas song, I hurt inside, realizing this
holiday season might be our last. When I went to Christmas
Revels at the University of Houston as I did every year with a
group of friends, a sudden premonition stabbed my heart. *Next
year when I come, will I be a widow?*

Widow. I hated that word. It connoted a dried up old lady
with a face like a prune, a squeaky voice, and a faltering step.
Mostly it meant "alone." I didn't want to be alone. I didn't think
I could bear it. At night I curled up close to Ralph, savoring
his body heat, the sound of his breathing, the substance of my
husband.

On December 10 we went for a follow-up visit to Dr. Riker.
He marched into the examining room. "Good morning, sir,
madam," he said crisply.

"Madam" was acceptable, I guessed, but "sir"? He'd been
my husband's doctor for well over a month. Surely he could
call Ralph by name.

The doctor sat down and pulled up the chart on the computer.
"You're in remission," he began.

"What does that mean, exactly?" I asked. "Will remission
last a week? A month?"

Dr. Riker looked annoyed as if it were not my place to speak.
"A month, perhaps," he answered with a shrug.

"The bone marrow people came to see me," Ralph said.
"I need to make a decision about a transplant. I want some
numbers."

Dr. Riker had no hesitation giving them. "You have a ninety-
five per cent chance of being dead in five years. With a bone
marrow transplant, even if the team decides you're eligible, you
have a seventy per cent chance of dying."

Not a five per cent or thirty per cent chance of living. Why did this loathsome man insist on stressing the negative?

"If I have a transplant, I'd like to do it after February first," Ralph said. "That's when I switch from regular health insurance to Medicare."

The doctor's lips turned down. "We don't make plans around Medicare," he said. "We do the transplant during the first remission if possible." He rose. "You'll have another round of chemo this month," he said, striding toward the door and opening it.

"I have another question," Ralph said before the doctor could escape. "About the other patients on the clinical trial I'm on. Most were in remission the last I heard. Are they still?"

Dr. Riker stopped in the doorway and shrugged. "It's too early to say if their remissions will last or won't." Government privacy guidelines, which I, too, had to follow in my speech pathology practice, absolutely forbid such conversations within earshot of others, but the doctor didn't seem to care. He made no move to shut the door.

"Can you give me the current information?" Ralph persisted.

"Sir, I honestly can't remember which protocol you're on."

The computer was three steps away. The doctor could have looked up Ralph's protocol, but he obviously considered it a waste of time. Ignoring me, he nodded at Ralph and disappeared.

I wondered if he treated his family with the same disdain he did his patients. I had an urge to follow him through the door and yell, "Go. To. Hell."

I made a mental note. I would add a chapter to my book: "How to Deal with Arrogant Physicians."

Still seething, I went downstairs with Ralph to the Ambulatory Care Center where he was due for a transfusion and left him typing on his laptop while blood dripped through the catheter.

I found one of the hospital's meditation rooms, went in and began to cry. Did Dr. Riker see us as people or lab rats? I expected objectivity, but this man seemed to take pleasure in telling brutal truths. Or perhaps he'd become so inured to cancer, he had lost any understanding of its emotional effects on patients and their families. I remembered my childhood doctor with his kind, quiet manner. So long ago. I wondered if this was what medical science had come to.

After the rush of tears, I dried my eyes. A stack of cards and brochures lay on a table. I picked up one of them. It was a poem, "What God Hath Promised," by Annie Johnson Flint. It began like this:

> *God hath not promised skies always blue,*
> *Flower-strewn pathways all our lives through...*

I certainly agreed with that. The poem wasn't Shakespeare, but it spoke to me. I hoped God, or Someone, would give me strength. I'd always gotten my strength from Ralph. Alone and storm-tossed, I needed something to hold on to. I took the card home and placed it beside my computer. For the rest of our cancer journey, it was my mantra.

♦♦♦

On the way home later, Ralph said, "Someone has to be one of that five per cent. Why not me?" His voice was cheerful, his hands steady on the steering wheel. That was so like him, always finding the positive, even if he had such a small chance of survival. And so unlike me, who always thought the worst.

"I don't know how you feel about your doctor," I ventured, "but I don't like him."

Ralph surprised me by saying, "Neither do I. He should have looked up my protocol."

"So you won't be angry if I call and ask for a different doctor?"

"Not at all," he said.

The next day I spoke to the social worker. "Someday I may have to be the one communicating with this man, and I can't. I have no doubt he is a fine research scientist, but he has no empathy. When he talks to a patient, he's like a robot. I don't expect him to be our pal, but I want a doctor who treats us with some care."

I wanted her to know I spoke from experience. "I've been seriously ill myself," I said. "I caught fire from a stove when

I was nineteen and was burned over thirty-five per cent of my body. My doctor was the head of plastic surgery at UT in Galveston and a consultant at Brooke Army Hospital in San Antonio. He was an incredibly busy man, but he always made me feel he was fighting for me, that he wouldn't give up. And the day I finally was able to walk into his office, he came out in the waiting room and stood there with tears in his eyes. That's what I want in a doctor, not an automaton who doesn't even know my husband's name." I was out of breath and near tears when I finished.

"I'll see about making the change," the social worker said.

We got our new physician, Dr. Kerrigan, within a week. I went with Ralph for his first appointment.

Another office like Dr. Riker's. Same white walls, same examining table, same view through the window, of other medical center buildings piled up like blocks. Please, not the same kind of doctor.

There was a tap on the door, it opened, and Dr. Kerrigan stepped into the room. His hair was ash brown, his face smile-creased; his khaki pants looked lived in. I'd heard he biked to work every day. He looked like the kind of guy you'd like to share a beer or watch a baseball game with.

"Ralph," he said and shook my husband's hand. He smiled at me – actually *smiled* – and sat down. He glanced at Ralph's chart. "I see you're doing well."

"I'm interested in knowing more about a transplant," Ralph said.

"Ultimately, that'll be up to the transplant department," Dr. Kerrigan said, leaning back in his chair. "Have you started the screening process?"

Ralph nodded and said he had more questions. "How much can I go out? I have a business; I need to see my clients."

"And," I added, "we'd like to go out to eat sometimes if we can."

"Just use common sense," the doctor said. "If someone at the next table starts sneezing or coughing, walk out."

Ralph asked a few more questions, we stood to leave, and Dr. Kerrigan high-fived him. "Keep up the good progress."

"We struck gold," I whispered as we started down the hall.

Ralph nodded.

I felt as if I were floating, as if I were in a balloon, wafting through the sky on a sunny day. We'd found a doctor with empathy, one who didn't make you feel you were stealing time from him, one who related to patients as people. Later I learned Dr. Kerrigan was recently diagnosed with lung cancer, but I imagine he'd always been a "patient's doctor."

Ralph went in for a couple of days for his second round of chemo. He came through it well except for an ongoing rash. He also insisted the food at the hospital tasted awful, no matter how impressively it was served, and as soon as he was in his hospital room, his appetite deserted him.

A few days later we celebrated our thirty-fourth anniversary with a quiet dinner at home. Silently, we held hands across the table and hoped we'd make it to year thirty-five.

On Christmas Eve morning I dropped Ralph off at the hospital, and later I went to Blockbuster to rent a movie. Going to a movie on Christmas Day seems to be a universal outing for Jews. A movie and Chinese food. "Why Chinese?" one of my non-Jewish friends once asked.

"Because Chinese restaurants are the only ones open on Christmas."

In our family, the annual Christmas Day movie was an event discussed and debated for weeks before Christmas. We liked to reminisce about past favorites: *Tootsie, Schindler's List, Shakespeare in Love*. This year would be different; we would watch the movie at home.

I rented *The Terminal* with Tom Hanks, walked out the door of Blockbuster and stopped at an amazing sight. Snow! A man about to walk in halted, too, and we both stared at the sky. Were those big white flakes drifting lazily down real? This was a logical question in Houston, Texas, which had not seen snow for at least five years.

I called Ralph. "It's snowing."

"Yeah," he said. "People here are standing at the windows gaping. The people from up north (anything above the Red River) think they're crazy." Ralph, being from Iowa, was not impressed with the snow itself, but the fact that it was happening on the Texas Gulf Coast was another matter.

The snow continued throughout the day. At midnight we pulled on our jackets and grabbed the camera. We raced outside into the chilly night and looked around to see a white sheen of snow on rooftops, a thin coat glistening on the grass and leaves. The night was so pure, so silent, so different from our usual holiday, it was nearly impossible to take in.

I want to rewind my life like a video and play that night again, feel Ralph's cold hand in mine, relive the joy.

A white Christmas in Houston, Texas. Even for Jews, this was an event for the ages.

CHAPTER 7

Ralph and I met at a Mensa party. I was a divorced single mom with two young children, beginning a Master's program in speech pathology. He was new to Houston, transferred from Kingsville by Celanese Chemical. He, too, was divorced and was about to get custody of Bryan, his three-year-old son.

This was one of my first ventures into the singles' world after a ten-year marriage. I'd forgotten the moves and the lines. I was as painfully shy as I had been in junior high. At the party, I wandered the room, then sat down and put on a fake smile. Before long, my lips hurt from the effort. I checked my watch. How long before I could escape?

A blue eyed man with a tall, gangly body and a crew cut approached me. "I'm Ralph Zirkelbach." He sat down beside me. Maybe, I thought, he felt sorry for me because I was alone.

This wasn't a "Some Enchanted Evening" encounter with our eyes locking across a crowded room. He glanced at me in passing and started a conversation. I was glad to have company. We chatted for a while and then he moved on. He was pleasant enough for me to decide the evening wasn't a total loss.

Years later he told me he'd thought I was interesting. I would have preferred sexy, charming, or at least attractive, but by then we'd been married for a long time. Maybe he'd forgotten what he felt that first night.

Being poor at remembering names, even one as unusual as Zirkelbach, I had no idea who he was when he called the next day. He reminded me of our conversation and asked if he could come by. "Sure," I said.

He asked me a lot of questions while we sat at my breakfast room table. "Is this an interview?" I inquired.

He laughed and asked me to go to a movie the next weekend. What the heck. He wasn't Jewish, but I figured he'd be good to practice on.

Thirty-five years later, I was still practicing.

◆◆◆

One skill I never mastered was how to get Ralph to open up about his inner thoughts. I knew he was not a man to talk about his emotions, his fears. Was his optimism about his chances of recovering from leukemia simply a well-practiced facade or was it real? Was his silence a way to protect me? I longed to reach into his mind, but he wouldn't share his feelings about his illness. And so, like him, I went about my daily life, concentrating on minutiae.

Now I wonder if I took the easy way out. Sometimes guilt wracks me. Why didn't I insist on talking about his illness and what it meant to him? Perhaps because I couldn't bear the burden of his fear. If I didn't ask, I didn't have to know. Other times, I realize no one could have forced this stubborn man to talk if he didn't choose to. Whatever secrets he harbored, he kept them inside.

I didn't speak about my own unending terror, for fear of adding my problems to his. Ironically, I had spent my life teaching youngsters to use language; yet I, the communication specialist, could not tell my husband what was in my heart.

Now I wonder, what if I had confided in him? I try to imagine what we would have said.

"I'm afraid."

"I'm not."

"I don't want you to be in pain."

"If I am, I am. No use worrying about it."

"I don't want you to be sick."

"Grow up, Thelma. It's not what you want; it's what you get. Besides, I'm going to get well."

And then he'd hold me close and I'd believe him – for a little while.

◆◆◆

The year turned. Sixty-six days had passed since Ralph's diagnosis.

On January 4, winter break over, I went back to work. On Mondays I saw children at a private school. I usually ate lunch there, but this first day back, I didn't feel like venturing into the teachers' lounge. I didn't want to hear the faculty talk about parties and winter vacations when I had spent my break tense with fear and worry.

I went home. On the counter between the breakfast room and living room lay some bags from Office Max, indicating that Ralph, now able to drive, had run some errands. I wandered into the bedroom and found him asleep so I tiptoed back into the kitchen and fixed myself lunch. Afterward I went back to check on Ralph.

Something about him worried me. His mouth was open, and it reminded me eerily of my mother's in the days before she died. I touched his cheek. His skin was burning hot.

"Ralph, wake up," I called.

"Huh?"

"Are you sick?"

"I dunno," he mumbled. "I went out before. I was fine."

"Let's take your temperature." I got the thermometer. His fever was 103.8.

"Maybe it's wrong. Get the other thermometer," he suggested.

This time, only minutes later, it read 104.2

"You have to go to the hospital. Call the emergency room and I'll get in touch with my office and cancel my afternoon appointments." My hands shook as I punched in my partner's cell number. She didn't pick up.

"Come on, let's go," I urged. "I'll call Karlene again from the car."

Ralph moved groggily out the door and got into my car. I tried my office again. Still no answer.

"Here's my patient list," I said to Ralph. "These two are my first kids this afternoon. Call and cancel them for me."

Ralph tried but I could tell he was making no sense. I grabbed my cell phone from his hand and took care of the calls myself.

I missed the turn to the Medical Center, the one I made almost every day, and had to keep going and make a U. When we got to the hospital, Ralph needed a wheelchair. He had long since changed from the skinny guy I first met. Six feet and over 200 pounds to my five one and 108, he was too heavy for me to push. I ran inside and got help.

We arrived at the emergency room and waited. And waited

some more. I watched the minutes crawl by, I watched the bored looking young man at the desk. I watched Ralph, and I wondered if he'd ever be called into a room. What if he just stayed here and died in the ER waiting room? Did that happen to patients?

He sat, oblivious to what was going on around us, which wasn't much. Every now and then someone would wander in with a patient, and they also would wait. The fear and frustration in the room were palpable.

Finally, after about forty-five minutes, a nurse called Ralph's name and led us to a small room. On the way we bypassed the triage unit, where critically ill patients were. Thank heavens we weren't going in there.

Once in the room we waited some more. Ralph's forehead was cooler than before but not enough. When a pleasant young doctor came in and examined him, she said he probably had an infection, not unusual in cancer patients. "Happens all the time."

"Why?"

She lifted a shoulder. "Sometimes these infections come from the patient's own body. His fever's already going down. Don't worry."

As if I could simply flip the Off switch on my worry. But at least, now I knew this episode wasn't unusual.

"We'll shoot him with some antibiotics, keep him overnight, and see how he does," the doctor said.

I felt much better, but we still had to wait, first for the IV, then for the hospital room.

By six o'clock I was hungry enough to leave and get something to eat. When I was a child, mealtimes were sacred; you did not shove a frozen dinner into the oven late in the evening because you'd forgotten to buy something to cook. You ate at 8:00 a.m., 12 noon, and 6:00 p.m., no matter *what*. Ralph often remarked that this routine was so ingrained in me that if we traveled across three time zones and came upon a clock that said 6:00, I would be ready to chow down on tiger meat for dinner even if I'd eaten a massive lunch half an hour before.

Unable to control my growling stomach, I trudged to the cafeteria, redolent with the smell of old grease. The first chicken salad sandwich I'd eaten before Ralph entered isolation had suckered me in, but the gourmet presentation went downhill after that. This evening's dinner was unappetizing looking beef in even less appetizing gravy. I wrinkled my nose and picked up a pasta salad, which turned out to be nearly inedible. I poured myself some iced tea and grabbed a slice of apple pie (Sweets Under Stress, my lifelong motto). The dinner made me feel sick. Even the pie wasn't up to my lax standards. I went back to find Ralph still waiting.

When at last a pleasant man from Transportation had wheeled Ralph's gurney through the labyrinthine halls to the tenth floor and I saw him settled in his room, I went home, barely making it before I went to bed, exhausted. Two days later Ralph was home again. I promised myself if he ever again had to go into the hospital unexpectedly, I would be calm.

And when it happened, I was.

◆◆◆

Ralph was soon feeling well and again able to drive himself to his frequent clinic visits for blood testing and transfusions. I was pleased that he could do this because I no longer had to alternate with Keith as his chauffeur. In the passenger seat, Ralph felt it incumbent upon himself to criticize my driving. "You know, you don't hold the steering wheel right," he remarked one day. "You should rest your palm against it. Don't put your thumbs on the other side."

"I've been driving since I was twelve and too little to see over the damn wheel," I huffed. "Don't start giving me lessons now."

What percentage of married couples criticize one another's driving? I bet it's huge. Obviously the serious nature of Ralph's illness didn't interfere with our ability to do that.

Ralph also disagreed with my choice of routes to the hospital, insisting my way got us into heavier traffic. And darned if he wasn't right.

Each time he returned from the clinic, Ralph regaled me with stories about the people he met: the family from the Middle East who had chosen this hospital because it was reputed to be the world's best, the young woman who brought snapshots of her rash-covered belly and passed them around. He thought her exhibitionism was funny; so did I. Perhaps others wouldn't, but people in the throes of illness often indulge in black humor. You have to find something to keep your spirits up; even the most macabre details of the hospital experience are fodder for laughter.

During January we received an e-mail from our friend Brad Silver, saying that his wife Marian had passed away. Ovarian cancer had finally gotten the best of her.

Marian and Brad had been our friends for many years. We'd met through our sons. Sean and Michael became best buddies when they were in the same home room in fourth grade. We often went out together as couples. Marian and I sometimes went to lunch, and Brad and Ralph talked computers to each other every few weeks. When our boys grew up and went away to college, our two families always met for a special dinner out during Christmas vacation.

At the memorial service friends spoke of Marian as intelligent, involved in current affairs, an athlete, a leader. For Ralph and me, the service was poignant. As we sat in the chapel, shoulders touching, with the afternoon sun glittering through the stained glass windows, I wondered if Ralph, too, would fall to cancer.

Although I would miss Marian, my thoughts always cycled back to Ralph.

CHAPTER 8

One Sunday I was home and Ralph was at the hospital getting one of his frequent transfusions when the phone rang. The Cancer Institute flashed on the Caller ID. If Ralph were calling, he'd use his cell, so it must be the clinic to tell me ... what? Trembling, I picked up.

"Mrs. Zirkelbach? I'm calling from Bone Marrow Transplant to tell you we got your husband's family's screening results."

I sat down.

"He has a one hundred percent match."

"Oh my God."

"The statistics came out perfectly. One sibling was a zero match, two were fifty percent and one was one hundred."

"Who was the match?" I asked, but somehow I already knew.

"His sister Catherine."

"She said she'd be the one."

As thrilled as I was, I felt a weird tingle. When Ralph spoke to his siblings, Catherine, his youngest sister and a devout Christian, said she knew she would be the donor, that she was certain the Lord wanted Ralph to have her blood.

Catherine was the fourth child of Barbara and Richard Zirkelbach. Ralph was the oldest, his sister Kate a year younger.

Sara was born five years after Kate.

Sometime after Sara's birth, their mother suffered a bout of rheumatic fever. "The doctor advised her not to have any more children," Ralph told me, "but when she'd felt better for a few years, she asked if she could consider another pregnancy. The doctor decided she was healthy enough and a year later she gave birth to Catherine." Louis was born a year after his sister.

When Ralph told this story about Catherine's birth, I was sure that Catherine had been destined to save her brother.

February arrived, and we waited to hear the results of Catherine's further testing. Would a transplant be possible? Obsessing over the side effects of the procedure, I both wanted and feared it.

Work was my solace. There I could forget for a few hours the fear and worry that surrounded us.

One Monday morning five-year-old Bethany greeted me, "How are you, Miss Thelma? Know what? I was sick on Saturday. My tummy hurted. I almost throwed up." She smiled. "I'm okay now."

What a change from her language a year ago. I remembered returning one day after I'd had a sore throat and Bethany remarking. "Miss Thelma, you was last day sick? And so me." It was gratifying to know that in spite of the stress that often overwhelmed me, I was still able to make a difference in a child's life.

◆◆◆

At last we heard that Catherine's test results were promising. She and Ralph even had the same B positive blood type. She made arrangements to come to Houston in late February for the stem cell donation. Meanwhile, Ralph was transferred from the leukemia department to bone marrow transplant, where Dr. Chandra Helm would be his chief doctor. We met with her and liked her immediately.

My February romantic suspense for Silhouette, *Stranger in Her Arms*, was released. I scheduled only one book signing at a small neighborhood bookstore. Willa, the owner, had always supported my writing career. I remembered a signing there that my obstetrician-gynecologist attended. He asked me to sign his book "To someone who knows about the aftermath of love and romance."

For this signing, friends and colleagues turned out, and Willa sold her entire stock of my books as well as some extra author copies I brought along.

Noticing the crowd, a woman wandered into the store and picked up a copy of one of my older books, *The Truth About Elyssa*. She frowned as she peered at the cover, a man and woman in a sexy pose. "Is it a true story, an autobiography?" she inquired.

I only wish it were my autobiography and I looked like that. "No, it's a romance novel."

She dropped it on the table. "I don't read *those* books" she announced and hurried out of the store.

Oh, well.

♦♦♦

Valentine's Day arrived and with it, the anniversary of Ralph's and my first date a week after we met at the Mensa party. He arrived that long ago evening bearing a Valentine card with my name, or his approximation of it, on the envelope: Thema.

He did eventually learn to spell my name, but his spelling was always abominable. For years he called Ginny, my secretary, to have her look up the spelling of words he wasn't sure of.

On our first Valentine's we went to a movie, "The Shoes of the Fisherman" with Robert Mitchum playing Peter, the first Pope. Afterward we went for coffee and discussed the movie, others we'd seen and enjoyed, and our newly single lives. Something thrummed between us, and I knew this wasn't just a date; it was a beginning.

On this, our last Valentine's evening, we stayed home. Ralph gave me a card with a quotation from First Corinthians: "Love bears all things, believes all things, hopes all things, endures all things. Love never fails." I framed it, and it still sits in my study on the shelf above my computer where I can see it every day.

On the day that celebrates love and lovers I wondered what brings two people together. In all the random movements of millions of people whose paths cross or who miss one another's trajectories completely, how did we happen to be in the same place at the same time? And why did we happen to have a conversation? What made him stop instead of passing me by? The same chance that brings one egg and one particular sperm together? Synchronicity? God's plan?

Except for our IQ's (To belong to Mensa you must test out in the ninety-eighth percentile or above.), we were opposites. Ralph was friendly; I am shy. He was mechanical; I am a klutz. Neither of us was athletic, but I follow sports avidly; he always managed to disappear during the Super Bowl or similar events.

More significant differences: He was conservative; I am

moderate-to-liberal. He was impulsive, liking to do things at the spur of the moment; I like *plans*. Once on a cruise vacation we discovered we would have an extra day in London. It was August, and England was having a heat wave. "Where will we stay?" I worried.

"Wherever."

"We need a place with air conditioning."

"We'll figure it out when we get there."

"No, no, no," I said. "We have to figure it out as soon as we dock in Dover."

We figured it out in Dover. Ralph found us a lovely hotel in Kensington, supposedly with air conditioning. Unfortunately, the staff did not know how to turn on the A/C. Ralph had to go up to the roof with them to show them how it worked.

Another difference between us: When Ralph cooked, he made up the recipes as he went along, and everything he made was delicious, from his Thanksgiving turkey to fried plantains to spicy dips. My dishes are tasty, too, but I follow recipes religiously, never deviating by as much as a pinch of salt.

Ralph was a procrastinator; I like things *finished*.

Our most fundamental difference was that he was Christian and I am Jewish. For most of our years together, this presented no problem. We joined a synagogue as a family. Ralph went to synagogue, teaching himself Hebrew during the long Rosh Hashanah and Yom Kippur services. We lit Chanukah candles, had Passover seders, sent our children to summer day camp at the Jewish Community Center. When his family visited, we hid the wine and said prayers before meals. In Iowa we went to church.

The Zirkelbachs never gave up hoping that I would convert to Christianity and be saved. Although Ralph was firm that they not witness to me, his mother devised subtler methods of proselytizing: leaving leaflets on the bed table when we visited them. I usually read them, but moved not one inch closer to conversion. But they kept hoping.

CHAPTER 9

As the day for Catherine's arrival approached, Ralph and I had our fiercest argument and frankest conversation. The argument began over his will. Timidly, I suggested he find it, his life insurance policy, and his long-term care policy. I didn't want to broach the subject of death, but I felt I had no choice. I knew where *my* documents were, but Ralph had hundreds of files. If he died, I envisioned myself searching them for days, months, years.

Ralph ignored my suggestion. I knew how his mind worked. If he didn't make plans for dying, he wouldn't die. Ralph attributed his good health to eating a lot of chili peppers and thinking positively. This didn't extend to far-out methods of combating cancer, but it certainly included denying the likelihood that his first doctor was right, that statistics were against him.

Several years before, I had a severe gastrointestinal episode and feared I had a tumor. As soon as this thought occurred, I began typing a list: daily tasks, whereabouts of documents, phone numbers of people to call. I could not understand why Ralph didn't do this. I didn't want him to die, but I wanted us both to be prepared.

Since Ralph had been ill, I hadn't pressed him on many issues. But now urgency ruled. How would I breach the granite wall of his resolve?

After a number of quiet pleas for him to get his affairs in order, the planner in me couldn't take any more. I lost my temper. I cried. I screamed. "I don't want you to die, but you *have to protect me.*" Finally he gave in and gathered the documents.

Once our tempers cooled, we sat together and, for the first time, talked freely about the transplant. Ralph said he felt sure about the transplant; it was his best chance. "But if it doesn't work, I'm not afraid to die," he added.

Now that he opened up about death, I didn't want to think of it. "I don't want you to die," I said, crawling into his lap. "You won't."

He stroked my hair. "I've never told you this, but I've always planned to convert to Judaism."

Neither of us ever tried to influence the other to convert. Although we talked about religion and even argued about it occasionally, conversion was off limits for both of us. "I just can't do it while my mother is alive," Ralph continued. "She would be devastated."

"I understand." I laid my head on his shoulder and breathed in his scent.

For months I kept his confession close to my heart. In my mind, I see us there in our living room, locked in a warm embrace, loving one another and hoping for a future that would not happen.

◆◆◆

Catherine arrived on February 18. She is a tall, lovely blonde with the sweetest, most serene smile I've ever seen. Religion is central to her life. She and her family spent a year doing missionary work in the Dominican Republic. They brought a young Haitian boy to their home to live for a year and consider him a son. She's a talented stained glass artist and she's also fun to be around. Instead of being just a tense preparation for the transplant, the next ten days were like a family party or summer camp.

Catherine loves movies. She brought a couple with her, and she and I went to see "Million Dollar Baby" and "Hotel Rwanda." Ralph couldn't go; movie theaters are a hotbed of germs. Not that he cared. Since he discovered the remote, he preferred to watch several movies on TV at the same time, switching back and forth between them.

Catherine loves popcorn and brought some bags of her favorite brand with her, so we snacked when we watched movies at home. She is a fan of "American Idol" and insisted we watch it and vote. One night we all curled up together on Ralph's and my king sized bed and watched "Monk," our favorite show, on TV.

We went out for dinner in the evenings, I took Catherine shopping at Chico's, my favorite store, and Ralph introduced her to his clients.

Catherine's visit gave her an opportunity to become close to her brother for the first time. When she was born, he was in high school and soon he left for college, so he was a distant figure in her life, who appeared only occasionally. She remembered that he would lift her high in the air or ruffle her blonde hair, but they spent little time together. Now they had a chance to really get to know one another and they took advantage of it.

So did I. Our visits to Iowa were often short and filled with so much to do that there was rarely time for long talks with my sister-in-law. This visit cemented a bond between us, one I'm sure will always remain.

Despite our enjoyment of her presence, we couldn't ignore the grim purpose of Catherine's visit.

She underwent various tests to check her health status: medical history, chest x-ray, EKG, and others. For several days nurses injected her with Neupogen, which stimulates stem cells to spill over from the bone marrow into the blood where they can be harvested for transplant. To her delight, she learned that her physician was a pioneer in stem cell transplant. Our cancer hospital had lured him from Germany.

As friendly as her brother, Catherine met other donors: a sister donating for her younger brother; a woman from Europe, the only sibling in a family of four willing to donate for her seriously ill brother; a family from Maryland who mortgaged their house and moved to Houston for nine months for the husband's leukemia treatment, which was successful.

Finally came the hard part, the actual donation. Harvesting of stem cells is called apharesis. Two IVs are used, one to collect blood and separate out the stem cells, the other to return remaining blood to the donor. An exhausting process, it takes up to four hours.

Catherine burst into tears when the nurse disconnected the IV's. She said she didn't know why, except that the process was so emotional for her, she couldn't stop crying. Afterward, she came home and slept for several hours. Two days later she gave a second donation. This one was easier; when she complained of weakness the doctor ordered a dose of magnesium and soon she felt better.

She had given her brother the greatest gift one can, a chance to live.

Ralph, too, was readying for the transplant. Medical tests, business decisions, discussions with his clients, instructions to his employees, finally a revision of his will. Time was like a roller coaster, crawling one day, speeding the next.

One night, while Catherine slept in the guest room, Ralph and I made love for the last time. Mindful of Catherine's presence, I stifled my cries. This echoed our first lovemaking, on my living room couch one long ago evening when Ralph came to visit and we put our three children to bed down the hall. We had to be quiet, so it wasn't a rip-off-each-other's-clothes first time; it was more like giggling high school kids in the back seat of the car with another couple in the front.

That last night as the specter of death loomed, we held each other close. With the whisper of his breath on my cheek, I realized then that I knew several months before his diagnosis that Ralph was ill. After more than thirty years together, I knew the geography of his body as well as my own – the play of muscles in his back, the length and breadth of his bones, the springiness of his chest hair, the pucker of his nipples. That summer, in the way a person long attuned to another can, I sensed something different – in his scent, the tension of his body. I didn't know or even imagine then what it might be, only that something had changed. I never voiced that thought. Even if I had, the disease was already entrenched, its hold on Ralph's blood too strong to deflect.

Friday night Ralph went to the hospital for a chemo treatment. His doctor warned that most patients got very sick from this strong dose and required hospitalization for several days. Catherine and I took him and saw him settled in a cubicle, then went to the airport to pick up Catherine's daughter Fay, a lovely copy of her mom, who came from Chicago to spend the weekend. We stopped back by the hospital for Fay to say hello to Ralph and went home to sleep. I made Ralph promise to call before he went up to a regular room as the doctor had predicted.

At 6:00 a.m. the phone rang. "Hi," Ralph said. "I'm done. Let's go out to breakfast."

"You're not sick?"

"Nope."

This had to be a good sign, the harbinger of a successful transplant. Feeling more lighthearted than I had in days, I pulled on a pair of jeans and a sweater and went to pick Ralph up. We ate at Le Peep, a restaurant in the Rice Village shopping area that specialized in breakfasts. Sitting across the table from Ralph, munching on a bagel and watching the few early risers wander into the cafe, I believed the future was good. Of course there'd be some hard times, but he'd weather them and be whole and healthy again. Realizing how close he'd come to death, Ralph would stop procrastinating. And I'd be satisfied with the normal, the ordinary. I would be stronger, too, for having lived through this ordeal.

How easy it is to tell yourself fairy tales and believe them.

The previous Sunday Ralph had taken Catherine to services at the Redeemer's Baptist Church, an African-American church whose minister was the brother of a close friend. This week the three of us, along with Fay, went to Lakewood Church. Under the leadership of Joel Osteen, this church had become one of the largest and most famous congregations in the country. They'd even purchased the Houston Rockets' former basketball arena, the Compaq Center, and were rebuilding it to house their enormous flock.

At the time of our visit they were housed in a large building on the north side of town. Traffic backed up along the road leading to the church. Throngs of people headed from the parking lot to the building and filled the auditorium.

I was not happy to be there. Not because of religious differences, but because I feared the crowds. Even though his blood counts were still up, Ralph was supposed to avoid large gatherings. We hadn't gone to a movie on Christmas, yet here we were, surrounded by hundreds of people. I'd tried to convince Ralph we should skip the visit and watch the service on television, but reasoning with him was useless.

We found seats near the front and listened to the choir, which sang loud and long and sounded to me as raucous as a rock group. I am not fond of rock music and I disliked this type of Christian music, with the choir members clapping and moving in rhythm, even more. The music in my synagogue is as different from this as The Three Tenors from The Rolling Stones.

Joel Osteen, Lakewood's famous pastor, was out of town, but three athletes spoke from the pulpit about their membership in the church. One speaker was David Carr, the handsome quarterback of the Houston Texans football team, who had spent most of his NFL career on his back due to the inadequacy of the team's offensive line. Carr told us his son had been recently diagnosed with juvenile diabetes and was hospitalized at Texas Children's. The presentation about his family coping with a serious illness seemed especially poignant to me.

As the service wore on, I glanced around uneasily at the crowded pews nearby. Was anyone coming down with the flu? An upper respiratory infection? A random cough sent me into a rush of fear as I imagined the germs catapulting toward Ralph like bits of shrapnel.

If he gets sick, I'll kill him.

Fortunately, he didn't.

That evening we celebrated Ralph's birthday a day early. He was sixty-five. We tried to make this a joyous occasion, with special foods from Eatzi's gourmet takeout store and a cake with candles for past, present and future, but the future would test all of us in ways we could not then imagine.

My heart hurt as I thought how different this was from my sixty-fifth birthday five years earlier. Ralph scanned my brand new Medicare card into his computer and I used it on invitations asking a dozen friends to a luncheon to celebrate a very special birthday. On my actual birthday we were in Paris, staying in a tiny hotel on the Left Bank in a room so small we had to suck in our breaths to pass each other. We strolled along the Seine, wandered through the Louvre, enjoyed an elegant French dinner at a posh restaurant.

A photo Ralph took that day shows me glowing with happiness, sitting on a bench in front of Notre Dame. The snapshot of Ralph's sixty-fifth birthday shows a tired man with slumped shoulders, whose pale, almost grayish skin hangs slack on his face. His lips are curved in a half-smile, but I see now that his eyes are sad.

CHAPTER 10

At nine in the evening of Thursday, March 4, Ralph entered the hospital to begin the transplant process. Stefan, the night nurse, got him settled in his room on the eleventh floor, which was occupied solely by transplant patients. Each large, comfortable room featured a Murphy bed for the caregiver, many of whom stayed with their family member twenty-four/seven. This would not be the case for us. We explained during one of our pre-transplant meetings with Ralph's transplant physician, Dr. Chandra Helm, that I would continue working – someone had to bring in an income – and would come to the hospital in the evenings.

In our marriage Ralph was the caregiver. Not that I was sickly; I just wasn't very independent. I was raised that way. My mother always made decisions for her two daughters and constantly reminded us that "Mother is always right." When I became a mother for the first time at twenty-five, I was astounded to find that rightness did not automatically come with the title. I was never certain I knew best.

Independence was not encouraged during my childhood. If anything, it was discouraged. Never the rebellious type and constantly brainwashed by "Mother knows best," I followed Mother's rules religiously. My sister and I did not learn to cook, clean, make choices. Perhaps Mother thought we would never grow up. Alas, when I did, I found life baffling. I clearly recall making a panicked call home early in my college career to find out how to send out the laundry.

With this background, perhaps it was no wonder that I depended on Ralph to take care of me: listen to my problems, fix computer glitches (After all, that was his profession.), change light bulbs, unstop the toilet. Our new role reversal was a major adjustment for both of us. During his two months at home after the first chemo, I got used to relying on Ralph again. But I reminded myself that I'd managed alone during Ralph's hospitalization. I'd even handled my mother's funeral. Maybe I was getting stronger.

◆◆◆

That evening in the hospital, the nurse wrote a large minus five on the whiteboard in Ralph's room. During the next four days he would receive massive doses of chemo to kill off his blood cells, then there would be a day of rest and on Day Zero he would have the transplant.

Then the real count would begin. The first hundred days are critical for a transplant patient. During this time the new cells engraft ... or don't. Tacrolimus, a strong anti-rejection medicine, defends the patient but can cause side effects. While the body acclimates to its new blood cells, all sorts of other difficulties can occur: lung problems, kidney problems, the dreaded Graft Versus Host Disease. Dr. Helm gave us a large white loose leaf binder with information about transplant and told us some doctors believe a mild GVH reaction is good; it indicates normal body behavior; other doctors believe no reaction is better. She herself ascribed to the "small reaction" theory.

I had no theory. I just wanted this to be over.

Ralph was calm, confident as usual. He noticed immediately that his room had a small alcove, the perfect spot for his computer and other office equipment.

We soon left his room to walk around the floor and get the lay of the land.

To make navigating its huge spaces easier for visitors the Cancer Institute was color-coded. The clinics were rose, the main hospital area was green and was accessed by the green elevators. The floor itself was divided into four wings; for the two on each side there was a family room with a TV, fridge, microwave, table and chairs. Not a particularly attractive or welcoming place, it still provided for many families relief from constant patient care.

Each nursing station had a large whiteboard with patient assignments written in blue marker. Because transplant patients require so much care, nurses were assigned no more than three per shift.

Between the rooms we saw sinks for staff and visitors to cleanse their hands with antiseptic. Cartons of masks and gloves in different sizes lay on the counters as well as boxes of yellow gowns. Some patients' door had signs, instructing visitors to don gowns. Inside each room was a large box for disposing of those gowns before visitors left so bacteria would not be spread to others.

Pictures of family members, friends, and pets adorned several doors. Others had instructions for the nursing staff: No Tylenol meant that the patient was being readied for transplant.

Beside each door was a sign with the patient's name and current doctor. "Current," because the Cancer Institute is a teaching facility. That means doctors rotate hospital duties, providing direct patient care for only two weeks every couple of months. Rarely is your clinic doctor the person you see in the hospital.

Rotation benefits doctors. One physician told me if he were constantly on call, he would never be able to fulfill his teaching duties; nor, I suppose, would he get many full nights of sleep.

For patients, rotation is immensely frustrating. And frightening. Getting accustomed to so many different doctors' personalities and styles of care, especially when you have a loved one in critical condition, is horrendous. Hospitalization denies you the control of your life. Being shuffled from one physician to another only compounds the feeling that you have no say in your own life, that you're in a maze, coming upon dead ends, trying to get out.

The only good thing is that when you get a doctor you don't like – and there are plenty of those – you know you'll get a new one in two weeks.

The physician you actually get each rotation depends on the luck of the draw. Even when Dr. Helm was on call, Ralph wasn't always her patient. So there's always the scary suspicion that the new doctor doesn't really know your patient's condition. One doctor reassured me that the staff met weekly to discuss patients so they were all aware of each one's needs. I could only pray this was true.

As we strolled through the hall that first night, a couple approached us. The husband, a man near our age with gray hair and bright blue eyes, greeted us with a wide smile. Holding on to her walker, his wife stared zombie-like into space. She was bald and emaciated with skin yellowed from jaundice.

The husband introduced himself. "I'm Henry Lederman,

and this is Sylvia." During our brief conversation Henry told us they lived in Michigan but except for a few weeks' respite, had been in Houston nearly a year. He nodded toward his wife. "She's had CML (chronic myelogenous leukemia) for thirteen years. Last year she had a transplant and now she has Graft Versus Host Disease."

Not what I wanted to hear at the beginning of Ralph's hospital stay. Was this the "life" Ralph had to look forward to? If so, would he want to live?

I swallowed hard as Henry said good night and gently urged his wife along. I felt drawn to them in some unpleasant way and was compelled to turn and watch them make their slow and painful way down the hall. Even as I stared at the almost mummified woman, I wanted to blot her image from my mind. I turned away and faced toward the future.

CHAPTER 11

March 9, Day Zero. The day of the transplant. Ralph's new birthday, Dr. Helm called it. I called it terrifying. We stood on a precipice, and today we'd make the leap into space. I'm a clinger, not a leaper, and all I could think was, *Where will we land?*

Amazing that the day I'd longed for and dreaded started no differently from any other. For the first time, I spent the night at the hospital. I woke in the morning to see a nurse checking Ralph's vital signs. Ralph chatted with her calmly.

I was calm, too. On the outside.

I wished him a Happy New Birthday and gave him a card that said, "Today is a gift, waiting to be opened." I signed it, "With love and hope, Thelma."

Then I went to the cafeteria for my first Franklin Cancer Institute breakfast. I spied an omelet station. What a surprise. Just like brunch in a fancy restaurant.

I ordered a cheese and mushroom omelet, hash browns and a biscuit. Second surprise: Cancer Institute cooks were capable of ruining an omelet, making it taste like it was a week old. How hard could it be, I wondered, to scramble eggs? Or maybe my fear made everything tasteless.

Back upstairs, we waited. In a hospital you get used to it. I kept glancing up at Ralph, wanting to say something memorable, but no words came.

Finally the nurse practitioner, a stocky man in a white coat, arrived, bearing a small plastic bag of what looked like ordinary red blood cells. He connected it to Ralph's catheter line and stayed to monitor Ralph's vital signs.

The blood dripped through the line and into Ralph's body, like a regular transfusion. No sounds, no smells, only the steady drip, drip, drip into the plastic tube. Shouldn't there be a drum roll or the blast of a trumpet?

Something should mark this IV as different, I thought. The blood should be redder, the rate of infusion faster. Or slower. I couldn't take my eyes off small bag that held such hope. I watched the cells trickle until, after thirty minutes, none were left.

The nurse disconnected the bag and left the room. That was all. The most important moments of Ralph's life – and mine – were over.

A knock on the door startled us. "Come in," I called, expecting a doctor or a nurse.

Instead, Lisa Bronstein, the tall, dark-haired Jewish chaplain who became a good friend to Ralph during his stay in isolation stepped into the room. "I see you've finished your transplant," she said. "This is a significant occasion. I'm going to do a ceremony."

Carrying a *shofar*, she walked to Ralph's bedside. Old Testament readers will remember that on Mount Moriah God sent a ram to Abraham to sacrifice in place of Isaac, his son. The *shofar* is a ram's horn that is blown on the most solemn days of the Jewish year: Rosh Hashanah, the New Year; and at the end of the service on the Day of Atonement. The slender, curved horn has an unearthly sound that speaks to the Jewish soul. Its long, piercing cry connects us to our people and our God. Here at last was our trumpet.

Lisa said a prayer, blew three blasts on the *shofar*, and together we read another prayer:

O Merciful One, open the gates of Your
wondrous storehouse, releasing
your sparkling dew.
Droplets of dew, come for a blessing,
not a curse;
Come for life and not for death.
Come gently, filling with peace the
reservoir of my soul.

Comparing blood to dew made it sound delicate. I wanted the cells that dripped into Ralph's body to be stronger, like warriors that would build battlements around his organs, defend his body. Still, I bowed my head, shut my eyes, and prayed in my heart of hearts that the words of the prayer would be true, that life, not death would come from this.

Do prayers work? I hoped so.

In his book *When Bad Things Happen to Good People*, Rabbi Harold Kushner suggests during illness or loss, one should pray for courage to face what must be faced, so that is what I did.

I never viewed myself as courageous, but thinking back, I realize I had made progress. I didn't fear being alone at night, nor did I feel afraid when leaving the hospital in the dark. My cousin asked me once if I was frightened walking through the shadowy, cavernous parking garage across the street from the hospital. "No," I said, "not at all." This was true, although the garage was often deserted at the time I left, usually long after the night shift staff who parked there came on and the day shift departed. I never saw a security guard at the garage entrance, nor did the lack of one bother me.

When I was burned at age nineteen and a patient for three months at John Sealy Hospital in Galveston, my parents took a room at a nearby motel. Each day my mother stayed with me until nine o'clock and then my father took over. Afterward Mother said that although she walked back alone in the dark through an unsavory part of town, she never thought to be afraid. And now I understood. My mind was on Ralph. He was all the mattered.

Now began the excruciating wait for the transplant to engraft. Every night before I fell asleep, I whispered, "Please let it engraft."

We studied Ralph's daily blood counts as if they were sacred texts. A sharp rise in counts would mean engraftment. What if that didn't happen? The possibility was too awful to consider.

How would I go on without Ralph? Without him, I'd be disoriented, lost. He was my compass.

After a few days, his hair began to fall out. I had dreaded this since his first round of chemo, seeing it as the ugliest and most noticeable sign of cancer. One evening when I arrived at his door, Ralph's head was shiny and bald. The hospital barber had shaved him that afternoon. I was surprised that I didn't mind his new look at all. I decided he was now a cross between Bruce Willis and Shaquille O'Neal. Of course, he didn't care one way or the other. Looks – or locks – were not high priority for Ralph.

◆◆◆

When I wandered the eleventh floor, I frequently ran into Henry Lederman. Sylvia was not improving, he told me. She was having special treatments daily. He looked tired but still upbeat. I envied him his optimism and courage. And his friendliness. Everyone knew him. If I met someone elsewhere in the hospital and mentioned that my husband was on the transplant floor, invariably I would be asked if I knew Henry Lederman. He was an inspiration to both patients and staff.

Meanwhile, Ralph became ill for the first time. He had pseudomonus, a bacterial infection. Because of this, I had to "gown up" each time I went into his room. Soon the routine became second nature: wash hands, don yellow paper gown, find box of medium sized gloves and pull them on, slip on suffocating mask. After one hour in room, take off mask and breathe freely.

Ralph felt weak. His appetite declined; he wanted only yogurt or sherbet. Worst of all, he lost interest in everything, even his beloved laptop. During his first hospital stay in the isolation room, he spent most days absorbed in his work with his computer. Now he rarely turned it on. He didn't watch television. When I arrived after work, I often found the newspaper still folded on his bed table. "Don't you want to look at the *Chronicle*?"

"Huh uh."

"I could find the comics for you."

"I *said*, 'No.'"

He barely spoke to me, even to answer a question, and then in monosyllables.

Was this normal after transplant? Would this behavior continue? I didn't like the new Ralph very much, and I feared the transplant had changed his personality in some basic way.

Or was it my fault? Was I doing something wrong?

Upset and anxious, I decided to make an appointment with a social worker. I trudged along the confusing maze of hallways to the rose area, where the social work office was located. The receptionist told me the bone marrow social worker (Every department had their own.) was not in that day. Did I want to see someone else? I nodded and she said she would page one of the other social workers and have her call.

I waited fifteen minutes and then the phone rang. The receptionist directed me to pick up the extension.

"What did you want to talk to me about?" the social worker asked in a businesslike tone.

"I'd like to talk in private," I said.

"What about?"

In every elevator at the Cancer Institute hung a framed copy of the Patient's Bill of Rights. High on the list was the right to privacy. This woman reminded me of Dr. Riker. Hadn't anyone on staff read the elevator sign? "Look," I said, beginning to lose my fragile hold on my temper, "I'm sitting in the middle of a waiting room. I don't want to go into it here."

"I'll come down, then." She did not sound pleased.

By the time she arrived, I wasn't sure *what* I wanted to talk about. My thoughts hopped about like fleas as I followed the squat, sallow-faced woman into a small beige office and sat across from her.

"What can I help you with?" she asked.

"I ... I'm worried about my husband. He's had a stem cell transplant, and ... um, I'm not sure what to do," I stumbled.

"I don't know that I can help you with *that*," she said, and I realized I'd made a mistake. Social workers at hospitals were not counselors like the social workers I knew in private practice. If I'd come in and said I couldn't afford to pay for meals in the cafeteria or I was from out of town and needed a place to live, she'd have happily helped me out. As it was, she was as befuddled as I was. "Have you spoken to your husband's doctor?" she asked.

"No, I'm never here when he makes rounds."

Her eyebrows shot up. "Bone marrow family members are supposed to be with the patient twenty-four/seven."

"You know what? I talked that over with Dr. Helm. Someone in this family needs to work, and it appears that's me. He's in a hospital," I said, warming to my argument. "Can't *they* take care of him?" To my embarrassment, I started to cry.

The woman nodded sagely. "I can see you're upset."

Her words came right out of the introductory social work manual. *Anyone* could see I was upset. I got up. "I'll find someone else to talk to."

"You should contact the nurse practitioner in the transplant department. She may be able to help you."

"Thank you," I sniffed and left her office. I cried all the way back to the eleventh floor.

Upstairs I called the nurse practitioner, Donna Olson, who met me in the family room. She listened to my questions and quickly allayed my fears. Not to worry, she reassured me. Ralph's behavior was perfectly normal.

Relieved, I went home that night and surprised myself by bursting into tears again. I was ashamed of myself for questioning Ralph's behavior. He was sick. He had a right to be cranky and non-communicative.

I didn't have the right to be cranky back.

For the first time in our thirty-four-year marriage, I asked myself if I loved Ralph enough. *What is love, anyway?* I pondered.

Nurturing? I'd been so over-nurtured in my life, maybe I hadn't developed the ability to nurture someone else.

Devotion? Yes, I knew without question I was devoted to Ralph, that my life centered around him.

Understanding? I always believed I understood him, but now I had to grasp a changed person, who might never be the same.

Sacrifice? If I were called to appear before the Heavenly Tribunal and God asked me if I would sacrifice my life for Ralph's, would I say yes? I searched deep inside, down in the shadowy place that was my soul. The answer lay there waiting, but I pulled back. What if it were "no"? What if I didn't love Ralph enough? Frightened of myself, of my thoughts, I turned them elsewhere and dried my tears. I never allowed myself to go back there again.

♦♦♦

Since I now knew my worries about his behavior were unnecessary, I set about thinking of ways to cheer my husband.

The first hundred days are so crucial for a transplant patient that everyone, nurses and doctors included, knows what "day" a patient is on. I decided to give Ralph a method for counting his days. I bought two jars and a package of bright-colored peanut M & Ms. A hundred candies went into one jar, and each day I transferred one to the second jar. I liked shutting my eyes, grabbing an M & M and seeing what bright color I'd gotten. I liked the satisfying plunk when it landed in the empty jar. Ralph was not feeling well enough to be interested but I was certain he would be when he got better.

When I mentioned the jars to another patient's wife, she gaped at me as if I'd landed from another planet. "What made you think of that?" she asked.

"I work with kids," I explained.

"Oh," she said but she clearly didn't get it.

I covered Ralph's hospital room wall with snapshots of us, of his Iowa family, of trips we'd taken, of our children and two grandchildren, and of his cat Tiki. There we were in our parkas, standing on the deck of the Marco Polo cruise ship as we sailed to the Antarctic Peninsula, there laughing at a family gathering, there in a field of Texas bluebonnets.

March and April mark the height of bluebonnet season in central Texas. If he'd been well, this would be the time for our wildflower safari. Every spring we took a day trip, traveling west along Interstate 10, searching for bluebonnets. Our route was all freeway at first, then just past Columbus we would make a right onto State Highway 71, which meanders from there to Austin along the Bluebonnet Trail.

The bluebonnet, Latin name *lupinus texensis,* is the Texas state flower. I don't know how residents of other states feel about their flowers, but the sight of bluebonnets turns a Texan's heart to mush. I remember being on a tour bus in Peru when someone spied mountain lupines and yelled, "Bluebonnets!" and the bus full of delighted Texans broke into applause.

On our yearly trips, we sped through the countryside, eyes scanning the fields ahead of us. Red-orange Indian paintbrush, pale pink primroses, delicate purple phlox, spiderwort – they were beautiful but they were not what we were searching for.

Suddenly we would see a field. No, a lake, an ocean of blue. A blue so bright, so intense, so perfect it could exist nowhere but Texas. A blue so lovely it put the sky to shame.

We would pull to the side of the road and park to savor the

view. Ahead of us families spilled from cars. The children ran helter-skelter into the flowers and frolicked like puppies while the father recorded the scene for posterity.

Our own cameras clicked. We took panoramic shots of the brilliant blue blossoms against the verdant meadow grass. My favorite scene, tacked to the wall in Ralph's hospital room, looked across the sea of blue to a barbed wire fence, where a lone mesquite tree laced in spring green raised twisted branches toward the cloudless sky. Behind the fence a couple of brown Santa Gertrudis cows grazed. A black and white border collie lazed in the sunshine.

On our trips, I always snapped a close-up photograph, though I had dozens in my album. I bent toward the tiny plants, each petal shaped like a sunbonnet, hence the name bluebonnet. Their stalks are thick, bright green. Like the inhabitants of their home state, they are sturdy and strong, straight and proud.

I inhaled the spring perfume of the fields, of the sweet and tender new grass, of the colorful wildflowers. The April sun, already foretelling a scorching summer, heated my back. Dragonflies buzzed annoyingly around me. A mosquito always managed to zoom in and attack my arm.

Glancing over my shoulder for oncoming cars, I grasped prickly stalks and quickly pulled up a bunch of flowers. Ralph shook his head at me. It's against the law in Texas to pick bluebonnets along the highways. Laughing, I would scurry back to the car, clutching my contraband bouquet.

This year there was no bluebonnet trip, and the following year my son and granddaughter would take me in Ralph's memory, but at least we had pictures to enjoy and memories to cherish.

Also posted in Ralph's room was a get-well note from our fourteen-year-old grandson Marco and a story that our granddaughter, Gabriella, six in November and half-way through kindergarten, dictated for Popo: "The Blue Cornfield." Decorated with pictures she drew for him, it occupied a prominent place on the wall.

The joy of my life, Gabriella lifted my spirits whenever I saw her. She was born on Thanksgiving and that seemed apt; I thank God daily for this energetic little imp. Tiny with long dark hair and huge, mischievous brown eyes, she looks to me as if she's stepped out of a fairy tale ... although she'd rather be Junie B. Jones, the character from her favorite series of books.

"So, what's new with Popo?" she asked in a very adult voice each time we got together, and I would tell her how he was getting along.

And she'd respond, "He's going to get better. *I know.*" And I hoped, with the wisdom of childhood, she did.

Hearing about Gabriella cheered Ralph, so when I visited, I talked about her. His lips curved into a gentle smile. For a few moments we forgot about leukemia and were just normal grandparents, enjoying the antics of the favorite person in our lives.

CHAPTER 12

On March 26, Day 17, Ralph's transplant engrafted. He marveled at the significance of the date. Purim – the Jewish Feast of Esther – and Good Friday both fell on that day.

Tears rolled down Ralph's cheeks when he saw that his blood counts had risen. Although I had cried many times since his first cancer news, today my eyes were dry. I felt exhausted, as if I had carried a heavy burden and had finally set it down.

Whether because of joy, relief, or a high dose of steroids, Ralph could not stop talking. Over and over he remarked about the Jewish and Christian holidays occurring together. I enjoyed the sound of his voice, even though it wasn't as strong or forceful as usual.

Late in the afternoon the door opened. Gowned and masked, the woman who entered was unrecognizable. "I'm Dr. Helm," she said, and my heart almost stopped. She'd told us we'd only see her if something was wrong. What?

Before I could ask, she said, "I came to congratulate you on the transplant."

Ralph thanked her and chattered amiably until she left. Then we looked at each other. We'd received the official word. Life would go on.

◆◆◆

Catherine, Ralph's beloved donor, sent a congratulatory letter. He handed it to me, I read the first sentence, and skipped to the end, then set the letter down. "I can't," I whispered.

... I thank God daily for the healing in your body and that I could be a small part of it.

... Why am I taking the time to write you this letter? Not because I believe I'm telling you anything you don't already know, but because I believe there is only One that can give anyone spiritual life.

Please meditate on these things carefully...

As I read the letter now in its entirety, I know how much I admire this truly devout woman, who I feel is as much my sister as Ralph's. I respect her for speaking out for what she believed was right, but when I first saw her letter, I was shaken. And hurt. And angry. Ralph had made a decision to be Jewish, if not as a convert, at least in his heart. And now, would he return to a religion he'd virtually abandoned? Filled with fear and doubt, I wondered if he loved me enough to resist the pull of his old beliefs.

That night I couldn't sleep. I twisted in bed, kicked off the blanket and pulled it back, checked the clock on my bedside table again and again. Would Ralph abandon me? I vowed to ask him whether he'd act on Catherine's letter the next day but couldn't bring myself to do it. Did I have a right to that question? Ralph's heart belonged to me. Did he owe me his soul as well?

I wished I could talk over my doubts with someone. But who? Not my children, who would doubtless tell me I was selfish to feel so hurt, or my sister who'd say I was foolish. Not my friends. The subject was too intimate to broach with any of them. The rabbi? A counselor? No choice seemed right. I struggled alone.

Each evening I sat at Ralph's bedside and stated at him, unable to say a word, wishing he would mention the letter. But he didn't. I imagined that Catherine and I were engaged in a struggle for his soul. I knew my battle would be fought silently. Like the transplant, this was a decision he'd have to make himself I could not implore him to be Jewish. Judaism is not a proselytizing religion, and even if it were I would not risk the question. What if I asked him to convert and he said no?

◆◆◆

As his blood counts rose, Ralph's strength as well as his cheerful outlook returned. Wearing his gown and mask as required, he began striding around the eleventh floor. When I walked beside him, I could hardly keep up. This pleased both of us.

We met other patients but no longer ran into the Ledermans. One day I asked Ralph's nurse if Sylvia had been discharged.

"She moved ... downstairs," the nurse said. Her reply seemed both evasive and ominous. I surmised that "downstairs" was not a good place. In fact, Sylvia was now in ICU. I never saw the Ledermans again.

I spent the evenings and sometimes all night in Ralph's room, reading. The hospital has a large, well-stocked learning center, and from there I checked out books on leukemia. *Transplant*, written by a young man who had been hospitalized at Sloan Kettering, inspired me to believe we could get through this trying time.

I watched the NCAA basketball tournament on Ralph's TV. Since my alma mater, the University of Texas, had won the Rose Bowl, I had high hopes that they would win the basketball crown as well. To my disappointment they didn't make it to the Final Four.

At home late at night I continued my notes for *Leukemia Wife*, adding comments about the sweet young nurse who took the time to chat with Ralph each time she came into his room, about the patient around the corner who was suffering from Graft Versus Host Disease and whose joints had become so stiff he could hardly move, about the difficulty of telling what position each staff member held because all of them except the cleaning staff and room service waiters dressed alike.

I also worked on the romance I'd now sold to Silhouette. The heroine of the story, which was eventually released as *A Candle for Nick*, had a ten-year-old son with leukemia. I now knew more about the disease than I ever wanted to know. Ralph, in his illness, had done my research. And I knew how my heroine felt. At one point I had her say, "I feel like one of those pioneer women. They survive the long trip in the covered wagon, work side by side with their husbands to make a home. Then a tornado hits or the horses die, but they just keep on keeping on." Me too.

Friends called, sent cards, and e-mails, called to chat with Ralph, brought food, did my grocery shopping, invited me to meet for lunch or dinner. Lori walked over during her lunch hour several times a week to visit Ralph. Michael and Bryan, both of whom worked farther away, called to keep up with his progress. My children, Lori and Michael, regarded Ralph as their father.

Lori was in first grade when Ralph and I met. After her initial disappointment at learning that he wasn't the kind of engineer who drove a train, she quickly bonded with Ralph. He became her sounding board, her confidante, her confessor. She trusted his opinions and valued his advice. Along with the children, there was Valerie, my cousin, who became my "other" daughter when she attended medical school in Houston. Now living across the country, she checked in with us regularly by phone.

♦♦♦

Ralph and I settled into a routine. He had blood drawn before sunrise, doctor visits in the morning, and vital signs taken throughout the day. I came to the hospital after work, usually bringing my meager dinner and eating in the family room, where I chatted with other patients' family members and then returned to Ralph's room to stretch out on the folding bed and talk or watch TV until we both fell asleep. As the days stretched into weeks, I no longer noticed the sights and sounds of the hospital. Hairless patients listlessly walking the halls, anxious family members, urgent pages for physicians – all receded into the background, unpleasant but familiar.

I became immersed in the case of Terri Schiavo, the unfortunate young woman who had been kept alive in a persistent vegetative state by her family, against the wishes of her husband and, he insisted, against those of Terri herself, expressed long ago. These two bitterly opposing sides now engaged in the last battle for the life of Terri Schiavo.

I resented the media's intrusion on what should be a private time, and yet I was as much a voyeur as the rest of the American public, watching endless replays of the emaciated woman's head and eye movements and hand flutterings. I watched in horror as the combat in the courts accelerated, as the U.S. Congress made Terri a political pawn. I sorrowed for her family with their every move, every tear, recorded and beamed around the world. And yet like others, I could not tear myself away from the TV screen.

I sided with the husband, certain no one should live a life like Terri's. Why keep a heart beating in a body and mind that no longer knew life?

As Terri's days wound down, I asked Ralph what he thought. My husband was a man with strong opinions on everything from what tires to purchase ("No contest: Michelin.") to the war in Iraq, ("It's the right thing for America to do."). Yet when I asked how he felt about the Schiavo case, he answered, "I don't know."

"But ..."

"I don't want to talk about it."

"Haven't you been watching ...?"

His expression darkened and he shook his head firmly. "I don't want to hear about it."

I shouldn't have asked. The topic veered too close for him to deal with.

Still I watched.

I was relieved for Terri Schiavo when she died at last on March 31.

When I arrived at the hospital that evening, Ralph said nothing about Terri's death, although it was reported endlessly on all the news channels. Since he had expressed such aversion to the subject, I didn't bring it up. We went for a walk in the hall, greeting staff and other patients, pausing to view the photos tacked on the door of a new arrival. Marching along next to Ralph, enjoying his improving health, I forgot about the Schiavo controversy.

I had no idea that several months later, I, too, would be faced with a decision, and choosing life or death would become more than a compelling story about someone far removed. It would be personal.

CHAPTER 13

Dismissal was almost upon us. Since Keith, the driver Ralph had hired several months earlier, was not available every day, I searched for someone to take Ralph back and forth to the hospital. Remembering my impression of the duties of hospital social workers, I got in touch with the bone marrow transplant department's social worker. "Ah," he commiserated, "finding a driver is a problem."

"Can you help me?"

"No, I don't know of anyone."

I eventually found a lovely lady through the want ads in the neighborhood newspaper, and I resolved not to seek out a social worker again.

Ralph left the hospital on Tuesday, April 11. His friend moved his file boxes and electronic equipment out, and I packed. To his suitcase I added thirteen drugs. Tacrolimus, the anti-rejection medication, Zyrtec for allergies, anti-bacterials, and others I can't even remember.

Several drugs were not yet ready when I went to the pharmacy, so I wandered to the family room to eat a sandwich while they filled the remaining prescriptions.

Our rabbi stopped in the family room to say hello. A tall, dark-haired, cheerful man, he told me he'd said a prayer for Ralph and wished us good luck and good health. Ralph later related that the young nurse who happened into his room listened to the Hebrew prayer, her face disapproving, and as soon as the rabbi left, she said a Christian prayer for Ralph.

We agreed that we welcomed any prayers. Nevertheless, the shadow of Catherine's letter remained in my mind, and it seemed that religious differences loomed larger in our lives.

I remembered an experience when I was hospitalized for burns. Growing up the spoiled daughter of affluent parents in a quiet, well-ordered home, I never imagined that life would deal me any blows. Two months before my twentieth birthday I got my first lesson, and it was a brutal one.

I was finishing my junior year at the University of Texas,

living on campus at my sorority house, going to fraternity parties, beginning my clinical hours in speech pathology. I was active enough in campus activities to be a candidate for Mortar Board, an honor society for student leaders with high grade point averages. Then, on Tuesday, March 29, my life changed.

The spring day was warm, and before we left for class, my roommates and I opened the windows in our room to let in the sweet scented breeze.

This was the kind of day when walking the few blocks to the campus was a joy. I wore one of my favorite dresses, dark, long-sleeved cotton with a wide black belt. Under it I wore a crinoline petticoat, the rage that year, which made the skirt stand out like the dresses of pre-Civil War southern belles.

Round-up Weekend, one of the major celebrations at the University of Texas, was coming up in a few days, and the campus was abuzz with anticipation. The excitement carried over to evening. A short time before dinner another girl and I stood in my room, discussing what we would wear that weekend. The window was still open, but a cold front had blown in, and someone had lit the space heater. I stood with my back to it.

Suddenly my friend cried, "Thelma, your dress is on fire."

I glanced over my left shoulder. Flames shot up from my skirt, gobbled the flammable crinoline beneath it.

I knew not to run. That's the first thing you learn during Fire Prevention week in elementary school. I ran.

Screaming, I lunged across the room. My legs were on fire, and I thought in surprise that it didn't hurt as much as I would have expected.

I was only nineteen, too young to die. I ran into the next room, yelling for my friend who lived there and woke a girl who was taking a pre-dinner nap. I felt my bladder empty. Behind me I heard shouts. Someone threw me down, and minutes later the housemother rushed in and rolled me in a towel. "Please call my daddy," I choked.

As two firemen carried me downstairs to an ambulance, I thought the worst was over. It was just beginning.

Hospitalized for three months at John Sealy Hospital in Galveston, I was in critical condition. I remember the nauseating smell of my own burned skin, the excruciating pain, the skin grafts, the movement of the striker frame I lay on when it was turned every four hours. I had three grafts, fourteen surgical debridements, and after the grafts had taken, sessions of agonizing physical therapy.

One Sunday my parents went downstairs to the cafeteria for lunch. I dozed, then suddenly awakened as a man's voice said, "How are you, young lady?"

Flat on my stomach, I couldn't see him. "Not very well," I answered.

"Shall I pray for you?"

I realized he was a minister. A Catholic priest had stopped by my bed once, and the two Galveston rabbis visited regularly, so I was accustomed to pastoral visits. Still, I felt I should be truthful. "Thank you," I said. "I'm Jewish."

I heard his indrawn breath. "You must believe in Christ to be saved," he said, his voice vibrating with intensity.

"But ..."

"Accept the Lord or you will die and burn in hell."

I'd already been through the fires of hell. I began to cry. "Please," I begged, "leave me alone."

I heard his footsteps die away, but the memory of that encounter has never left me.

◆◆◆

For the moment, I shut religion out of my mind and focused on Ralph's homecoming. Life would get better now.

I went across the street to get the car. Spring had arrived while Ralph was hospitalized, and the roses in the Cancer Institute's garden were blossoming. I don't know who donated the garden, but I thanked them every day as I passed and inhaled the delicate perfume that reminded me of my mother's rose garden along the driveway in my childhood home. Although I missed the bluebonnets this year, I had the roses for company each day. Their vibrant colors atop thorny stalks seemed to embody a message that beauty and life could emerge from the horrors of cancer. On that day I believed it with all my heart.

As soon as we arrived at our house, Ralph went to his home office, the hub of his life. Seated before his computer, eyes focused on the monitor, fingers racing over the keyboard as if he were caressing a beloved's body, he looked truly at home.

His cat Tiki trotted into his study and perched on top of his TV, her favorite spot. Tiki was a slender gray tabby with a pretty face, large green eyes that gazed at the world with a serious expression, and a habit when petted of arching her back higher than any cat I'd ever seen. She was nine months younger than Toby, my furry tuxedo cat, and spent the first week after we adopted her in the fireplace, staring timidly through the screen at the comings and goings of us and our other cat. Then she came out and took over.

Tiki was the latest of a long line of Ralph's cats. She replaced his beloved Hal, who arrived in Ralph's life like a gift from heaven.

At that time Ralph's office occupied our garage turned game room. One day he heard a tiny squeak and found a three-month-old kitten in the desk drawer he'd left open the day before. He concluded that the frightened little creature had dropped through a hole in the ceiling. The cat was scared but he was a fighter, and Ralph had to don garden gloves to rescue the feisty, wriggling kitty ... and prevent the papers in his drawer from becoming cat litter.

The orphaned kitten lived in a cat carrier on the patio until Ralph tamed him and took him to the vet for shots. Because he'd arrived in our lives in October, we named him Halloween and called him Hal.

He was beautiful, with dark, wide stripes like an ocelot. He never lost his feral streak and though he managed at last to fit into our household, he did not enjoy being held and was terrified of the doorbell. I have a scar to prove that.

Once he moved out of the cat carrier, Hal remained on the patio for a while and had frequent encounters with our orange cat, Pumpkin, who was legendary for his friendliness. We decided that Pumpkin was teaching Hal social skills. Eventually Hal moved into the house and into Ralph's heart.

Of course, Ralph maintained that our pets were "only cats." They were nice to have around, but replaceable. But when Hal suffered his last illness and became so weak he couldn't move, Ralph was devastated. On the afternoon he took Hal to the vet

to be put to sleep, he sat in his favorite chair, ger
frail cat. His eyes filled with tears, and he said to .
picture." I look at it now, remembering the tender "toug-
who loved his cat enough to cry.

◆◆◆

The day after Ralph's homecoming I dropped him at the
hospital for blood tests and hurried to our synagogue school.
It was Young Authors' Day, on which children's authors, most
of whom were Jewish, were invited to the school to give talks
about writing and to autograph their books. I was scheduled to
speak to parents during lunch about my writing career.

That morning I sat at a small table across the gym from the
children's authors, watching with interest as the kids excitedly
bought books to be signed. Later, one of the children I worked
with said sadly, "Miss Thelma, no one bought your book."

"That's okay, Kenneth," I answered. "My books are not for
children."

At noon I did sell most of the copies I'd brought. I spoke
to parents and some of the teachers about genre writing, about
the fact that romance is the only genre in which the heroine is
as strong and important as the hero, not just an "object" for his
sexual desires. I told them that romance speaks to our needs
for intimacy and the universal drive for the preservation of
the species. I also spoke about my own journey to romance
publication, beginning by becoming a romance reader as I
traveled back and forth to Austin on the bus to visit my ailing
father. "I became a romance writer because I don't drive on
the highway." I talked about the thrill of selling my first book,
"second only to giving birth to my children," and about the
book I was writing now. I didn't add that I found romance
an antidote to the fears that pervaded my life, that as I wrote, I
let myself believe that Ralph and I, like the archetypal romance
hero and heroine, would live happily ever after.

As soon as I finished my talk and signed books, I hurried to the
hospital to pick up Ralph. Although he was clearly exhausted,
he wanted to know how my speech had gone. "Good," I said
and he smiled and reached over to squeeze my hand.

CHAPTER 14

Now that he was home, I expected Ralph to return to normal, but he had no appetite and very little energy. His appointments at the clinic wore him out, and he began running a low-grade fever. Nine days after his release he called me from the clinic to tell me he was going back into the hospital.

I wasn't worried. The nurse practitioner told us fifty per cent of transplant patients are re-admitted.

Ralph had pneumonia. The doctor started him on medication to combat the infection and drain off the fluid in his longs. Within a week he lost twenty pounds that he'd gained from fluid alone.

♦♦♦

The Saturday after Ralph entered the hospital Passover, the eight-day celebration of the exodus from Egypt, began. The first evening, Jews recall the escape from bondage during a ceremonial meal called the *seder*. The youngest child asks four questions, beginning with "Why is this night different from all other nights?" and everyone replies, taking turns reading the *Hagaddah*, the book containing the ceremony.

The *seder* meal is memorable: the cardboard taste of *matzoh*, or unleavened bread; the bite of horseradish, the sweet *charoset* made of chopped apples, nuts, and cinnamon; the cough-syrupy taste of the four cups of Manischewitz wine; parsley dipped in salt water, hard boiled eggs.

I remembered the Passovers of my childhood. My mother had rebelled from her ultra-Orthodox upbringing, but she always kept Passover. Special dishes, silverware, and utensils never touched by leavening, were kept in cabinets high above our kitchen counter. The day before the holiday Mother climbed on a ladder to get them down. Then she washed them with scalding water and put them in the lower cabinets which she'd cleared of our everyday dishes. The big green china bowl with a yellow border, in which she mixed ingredients for sponge cake, is part of my Pesach memories.

Daddy conducted the *seder*. I can see him now in his hat, holding a wine cup aloft as he chants the prayer, "Blessed art Thou, Oh Lord, King of the Universe, who hast created the fruit of the vine."

Jewish men cover their heads with skullcaps called in Yiddish *yarmulke*, in Hebrew *kippah*, when they enter the synagogue, eat, or pray. My father always wore his everyday hat. For me, his hat symbolized my father. When he died, I asked if I could have the hat he'd worn to the hospital. It was new, the price tag still in it: all of twenty dollars!

The hat sits on a shelf in my study. I like to rub the felt against my cheek; it's soft, like my father's voice. He barely spoke above a whisper but his words communicated authority. He taught me the importance of honesty, integrity. He taught me that your word means something; your reputation is priceless. "Stand up for your rights," he would say. "Don't be a quitter." He was my personal hero, the parent who loved me unconditionally.

Daddy was a small man, about five foot seven, but a determined one. He left the Ukraine at age eighteen to journey to America and join his siblings who had come before him. With no English and lacking an American education, he made his way, like many Jewish immigrants, by peddling. A photograph in the "Jews of Texas" exhibit in the San Antonio's Museum of Texan Cultures shows him with his wares in a horse and buggy. As always, he's wearing a hat.

Eventually he and a partner opened a service station. They each had a fifty per cent share, but Daddy was the boss. He worked long hours, especially during World War II when help was hard to find. He collected tires for the war effort, and a picture in the *Austin American* newspaper shows him standing beside a pile of tires higher than the roof of the station.

Despite his heavy work schedule, he always came home for lunch, washing his hands with Lava soap before joining the family at the table. In the summers, he made iced tea and I always wanted him to "fix" mine because I was convinced that nobody could mix in the sugar and lemons better than my daddy. Besides tea, he loved soft drinks. When he first visited my mother in Omaha, they stopped for a snack and he ordered a Dr. Pepper. Having never heard of the famous Texas soda, my mother thought he was ill.

He was highly respected in the Austin community, both Jewish and Christian. Although his first name was Alex, everyone called him Mr. Alec.

When I was in high school, I loved taking my friends to buy gasoline (19 cents a gallon then) at the station. My best friend still remembers the slogan: "D & S: High Test Gas for Less. We May Doze but Never Close."

As busy as he was, Daddy always had time to listen to my troubles and concerns. This year as Passover approached, I missed him more than ever.

◆◆◆

Several days before the holiday, an announcement arrived from Room Service, saying that the hospital would have special Kosher-for-Passover meals for Jewish patients and families. Ralph, still disinterested in food, didn't want anything, but I selected an entree and *matzoh ball* soup, chicken soup with fat balls made of *matzoh meal* floating in it. There would be no *seder* for us that year, but my mouth watered as I looked forward to the dinner.

A knock on Ralph's door signaled the arrival of my meal. I would eat in the family room because family members were not allowed to eat in transplant patients' rooms. I wished Ralph a *"gut yom tov"* a happy holiday, and hurried down the hall to begin my meal. The entree came, as I expected, in a Styrofoam container, since hospital dishes are *hametz* (used for bread) and using non-china dishes ensures they are *pesadich* (Kosher for Passover). What I didn't expect was a can of *matzoh ball* soup, sitting unopened on the tray. I stared at it a moment while the room service attendant beamed at me. "Um, how do I open the soup?" I asked.

"With a can opener." She looked at me expectantly, as if I might be concealing one up my sleeve. "Don't you have one?"

"No, I don't usually bring can openers to the hospital. And even if I could open the can, how would I heat up the soup?"

Ah, this was an easy answer. "Right there." She gestured

toward the microwave.

She thought I should put a metal can in the microwave? "Look," I said, "I don't want the soup any more. Just take the two dollars off my bill."

"Oh, yes, yes." She handed me back far too much money for the can of soup and when I tried to refuse it, she wrung her hands. "It's yours," she said and scurried away, leaving me to my lonely meal.

Seders end with the words, "Next year in Jerusalem." Throughout the Diaspora, the holy city always lodged firmly in the Jewish heart. Even now, more than fifty years after the birth of Israel, Jews still long for Jerusalem. But this year I changed the ending to "Next year in Houston." Ralph was recovering from his bout with pneumonia and the doctor said he'd probably be discharged in another week. I had every reason to believe that in 2006 Ralph and I would celebrate Passover at home with the rest of our family.

For the remainder of the holiday, I declined any further Passover meals from Room Service and brought my usual Passover fare, a peanut butter and jelly *"matzohwich."*

"You sure do like those crackers," observed one man in the family room.

"Not so much," I said. "I just have to eat them."

CHAPTER 15

April 28, Day 50, post transplant, began like any other day, at least any other in that surreal year. No premonition, no peculiar feeling. Nothing to warn me this would be the day on which our world would once more shift.

I arrived at the hospital around 11:30 that morning, managed to snag a spot in the always crowded garage, and found Ralph sleeping. He hadn't taken his morning meds and I shook him gently and reminded him.

"Give me a minute," he muttered and went back to sleep.

I gave him an hour. I'd begun attending a lunch group for caregivers called "I Have Feelings, Too." There I met people from Florida, Montana, Alaska, and of course from Houston, and heard their stories.

When I returned to Ralph's room, he was asleep and the pills still lay in the paper cup on his tray. "Ralph," I said, annoyed, "wake up and take your medication."

He didn't open his eyes. "Give me a minute."

I went out to the nursing station and told his nurse he seemed unresponsive.

"The doctor's already seen him today," she replied. "She said he's doing well and his vital signs are fine."

Unconvinced, I went back and sat by the bed. Every now and then I tried to rouse him, and each time he gave the same reply.

The physical therapist came in. "Mr. Z, I'm here to help you with your exercises."

"Give me five minutes."

The therapist looked at me. I shrugged. "I don't think he's going to cooperate," I said. "Maybe you should come back tomorrow."

Alone with Ralph I repeated the nurse's reassuring words to myself, but they didn't alleviate my concern. She may have believed he was fine, but the patient in the room wasn't Ralph; he was an unresponsive lump lying in the bed. The lunch I'd eaten downstairs sat heavily in my stomach. There's a "knowing" inside, no matter what anyone says, when your loved one is in danger. All wasn't well.

But what to do? Indecisive, I sat and stared at Ralph, willing him to wake up. Since he'd become ill, he'd handled discussions with the medical staff and decisions about his treatment on his own, and I always deferred to him. When my father was sick, Mother took over, speaking to the doctor *about* him. I vowed I'd never do that, but now I wasn't sure what I should do.

A technician knocked and came in, wheeling a large machine. "I'm here to take an echo cardiogram."

"Why?"

"His doctor ordered one, just to be sure everything's okay before discharge on Monday." She set up and began the procedure. Ralph seemed unaware of what was happening. Even when she asked him to move or turn to the other side, he barely responded, and she had to help him.

Frantic by now, I marched into the hall and insisted the nurse come in and check him. His vital signs were normal. "But he's acting strange." I protested. With a resigned sigh, the nurse agreed to page the doctor.

I was pleased at my unaccustomed assertiveness. I had been firm but nice. Nice was important. My hair-trigger temper was a lifelong concern for me. I would explode like a volcano, then my rage would evaporate like smoke, and I'd no longer be angry but ashamed. When I lost my temper as a child, my mother would warn, "Someday your face will freeze like that," or worse, "You should be like your cousin Beth. The sweetness shines out of her face." Meaning, "The temper shines out of yours."

But today I'd handled the situation appropriately. Within five minutes the attending physician's fellow, a physician doing advanced work, hurried into the room.

She examined Ralph thoroughly. She, too, was unable to rouse him. Before I could ask her what she thought was wrong, she strode out the door to the nurses' station.

In a few minutes she returned, this time followed by the nurse and Dr. Draper, the current attending physician, who performed her own examination while I stood by, waiting for her verdict, trying not to cry.

"We don't know what's going on," she finally said. "He may have an infection. We're going to start him on a different antibiotic." She followed the nurse to the door. "Don't call the pharmacy," she ordered. "Send someone down to get the drugs, *stat*."

I pulled out my cell phone and managed to key in Lori's phone number. "Something's wrong," I whimpered.

"I'll be right there," she said.

Dr. Draper, whom I liked for her pleasant, yet businesslike manner, said, "We'll do a C-T scan tonight and a lumbar puncture in the morning. The leukemia may be in the spinal cord; if so, it won't show up on a bone marrow aspiration. The spinal tap will tell us. Or he may be getting encephalitis."

I sank into a chair. Ralph had the transplant, it engrafted; now we were supposed to live happily ever after. Leukemia of the spinal cord? Encephalitis? They weren't part of the plan. The big white book about transplant that Dr. Helm had given us didn't mention these things in its long list of complications.

Out of breath, Lori rushed into the room. She must have run all the way from her office at Baylor. She took a look at me and went pale.

Dr. Draper acknowledged her with a nod and leaned over Ralph. "Mr. Zirkelbach, do you know where you are?"

"Huh ... uh."

"Do you know what day this is?"

"Gimme a minute." His speech was slurred, and this frightened me even more. Had he suffered a stroke?

"Mr. Zirkelbach, open your eyes. Your wife is here. Do you know her name?"

Ralph opened one eye. He barely focused on me, but finally mumbled, "Thel...ma."

Dr. Draper turned to me. "If you'll go out to the nurses' station, you can sign the papers to okay the tests."

Urgency made me stumble as I hurried out of the room. At the counter I picked up the consent form and scanned it. Complications of lumbar puncture: severe headache, back and/ or leg pain. Less common: puncture of the spinal cord.

Every medical procedure, every prescribed drug has a list

of possible complications. And Ralph was in the number one cancer hospital in the world.

I picked up the pen and signed my name. And plunged us into the Valley of the Shadow.

CHAPTER 16

I returned to Ralph's room to find people bustling around. "We're moving him to the wing on the other side of the building where they can put him on a monitor."

I packed his things, tossing them into the white paper bags the hospital provided and that seemed to multiply in our room. Thank heavens he hadn't been here long enough to amass his usual array of computer equipment and office supplies.

I suppose that sometime I went downstairs to eat dinner. I can't imagine failing to eat.

Early in our marriage, we drove to Iowa to visit Ralph's family. He decided we would spend the night in Oklahoma City. We arrived late, checked into a motel, and finally around 9:00 trudged into the restaurant. By the time our dinner was served, it was 9:30 and I was shaking with hunger. "Don't ever make me wait that long to eat," I told Ralph as we headed back to our room. And he never did.

After my hospital "dinner," I went upstairs to find Ralph still unresponsive. Later, he was taken downstairs for a C-T scan. Because his immune system was low, we waited inside a glassed-in room for the technician to come. The regular waiting room, occupied only by a woman at the desk, was dim and silent. I clenched my hands as tight as I could and wondered what the scan would show. Encephalitis, leukemia of the spinal column, a stroke?

The results of the scan were unavailable that night. Lori and I trailed Ralph's gurney upstairs. She went home, and I pulled down the Murphy bed and tried to sleep. During the night I woke several times to the sound of Ralph talking to the nurse, telling her he had to go to the bathroom. He was conscious, more alert. Relieved, I fell back to sleep.

In the morning I found him feeling better, so I dressed quickly, drove home to feed the cats, and went to the school at our synagogue. I had only one appointment on Friday mornings so I felt comfortable keeping it and driving back to the hospital. But when I arrived and walked down the hall to Ralph's new room, I heard him shouting. "No, no, no!"

Hands shaking, I grabbed a gown, mask and gloves and pushed open the door. A group surrounded the bed: the fellow, several nurses, an aide.

"What's going on?" I asked in a strangled voice.

One of the nurses turned. "They're trying to get him to allow the lumbar puncture."

I stepped forward. "Ralph," I begged. "You have to let them do this."

"No."

"Please. They need to find out what's wrong."

"No!"

Helplessly, I looked at the nurse.

The fellow raised her voice. "Mr. Zirkelbach, do you know where you are?"

No answer. I leaned against the wall and sobbed.

"Mr. Zirkelbach, how old are you?"

"Don't know."

"Please. Turn over so we can do the spinal tap."

"O...kay."

I shut my eyes. I didn't want to see, but I could hear. "No," the fellow said. "Can't get the needle in. Not quite," she said again. "I'll try one more time." I held my breath. "There, I've got it."

After a minute, I opened my eyes and saw her step away from the bed. The nurses disappeared, and I walked to Ralph and held his hand.

"Thelma?"

"I'm here. They're finished."

"Okay." He fell asleep.

Near noon Ralph awoke, moaning. "Hurts." His voice cracked.

In the six months of his illness, he'd never complained of pain. I jabbed the call button. The nurse came in and said pain wasn't unusual after a spinal tap and he could have medication. After a while, the pain subsided, and Ralph slept peacefully.

That evening I debated whether I should go to my writers' critique group. My book deadline was coming up and we met only every other week. I asked the nurse if I could leave.

"Oh, sure," he said. "He's okay. Tell you what, give me your cell phone number. We'll call if we need you."

As I drove away, I felt uneasy. Still, I kept going.

Why didn't I turn the car around? Even now I'm ashamed that I left Ralph that evening.

I wonder if I fled because I couldn't face his agony. Later I would have to watch him suffer, but this was still early in our journey, his pain still new. Or was I plain selfish, putting my book before Ralph?

At nine o'clock, as my critique partner and I chatted, my cell phone rang. I yanked it out of my purse. "Mrs. Zirkelbach, your husband is complaining of pain again, but he can't tell us where he's hurting. Maybe he'll tell you."

I heard him moaning in the background. "Let me talk to him," I said.

Ralph mumbled a hello and moaned again. I felt his pain in my own bones. "What's wrong?"

He didn't respond.

"Please tell me where you hurt."

"My groin."

I told the nurse and added, "I'm on my way back." Filled with self-disgust for having left him alone and in pain, I stuffed my papers into my bag and dashed to the car. The drive to the hospital was forty minutes ... or hours ... or weeks. I drove in a daze, barely aware of traffic on the freeway.

When I reached Ralph's room, the door opened and Bryan emerged. "How's your dad?" I asked.

"Sleeping. They gave him some medicine for pain."

Thank God.

"He said this morning they stuck a needle in him."

I nodded and explained what happened and why the spinal tap was necessary. "But he's better now," I said, more to encourage myself than Bryan.

"I'd better go," he said and took a step down the hall.

I watched him walk away, and then gowned up and tiptoed into Ralph's room. It was dark, but I could hear his deep, steady breaths. Reassured, I undressed quickly and lay down. Spinal taps cause pain but it's temporary, so I was certain we were over the worst. Ralph would be back to his old self in the morning. I curled on my side and let the dark lull me to sleep.

The next morning I woke to find Ralph clear-eyed and lucid. "Are you feeling better?" I asked. When he nodded, I said, "I'm going home to feed the cats. I'll be back soon."

At home I indulged myself in a carbohydrate-heavy breakfast – muffins with strawberry preserves – lingered over the newspaper, and took a long, refreshing shower. How I enjoyed the privacy of my own bathroom. When I spent the night at the hospital and showered there, I was always afraid a nurse or aide or even a cleaning person would walk in on me. Plus the shower in Ralph's hospital room was tiny and the small bathroom doubled as a storage room for extra linens, so I felt claustrophobic there.

This morning I was more relaxed than I had been in several days, and there seemed no compelling reason to rush back to the hospital. Doctors made rounds later on Saturdays, Ralph was back to normal, and I needed these precious minutes for myself. I petted Tiki, rolled an ice cube across the room for Toby to chase (his favorite pastime) and sipped a second cup of tea.

Driving back to the hospital, I listened to "Car Talk." Ralph had introduced me to the radio show during a drive to San Antonio. "Why would I want to hear about auto repair?" I grumbled when he mentioned the program.

"Just listen," he said. "You'll like it."

He was right. The show with the two car experts from Boston became my one of my favorites, too.

At the medical center I parked in the garage, strolled across the street and up to Ralph's room. "Hi," I said as I opened his door. "Feeling o ...?"

His scowl stopped me.

Tension crackled in the room. "Something's wrong," he said.

Not the same thing as yesterday, I thought, noting his clear voice and sharp eyes. I glanced at the monitor. All the numbers looked normal. "What?" I asked.

His jaw clenched, his hand stabbed the air. "I can't move."

"But ... but you *are* moving. I can see ..."

"My legs, dammit."

Was he losing his mind again? No, he seemed much too alert. And far too angry. He must be mad at the doctors for all the pain he'd suffered and was probably exhausted from the effects of the drugs they'd given him. "You're weak from all that's gone on lately," I told him.

'Look at my legs," he ordered. "Pull back the sheet."

I did. He tightened his fists, grunted, strained. Nothing happened. No movement, not even the slightest twitch of a toe.

No, this couldn't be happening.

"I showed the nurse," Ralph said. She paged Dr. What's-Her-Name."

"Draper," I answered automatically, still unable to process what my eyes saw. The word "weak" stuck in my mind. "Paralyzed" did not surface that morning, was not allowed to.

A brisk knock sounded and Dr. Draper entered the room, trailed by the fellow. They examined him.

I stood where I was, staring blankly at them, trying to remember all I knew about leukemia. A blood cancer. Nothing Dr. Helm said, nothing in the book she gave us mentioned leukemia affecting the nerves. But Ralph had had neurological symptoms the other day. Had he developed a new disease?

Dr. Draper finished her exam and stood back. "It's likely a hematoma that formed in the spinal cord and is pressing on the nerves."

Stunned, I could whisper only one word: "Why?"

"The lumbar puncture must have caused it."

But that wasn't one of the side effects listed on the paper I'd signed...

The paper I'd signed. No, no, no.

Ralph's face reddened. He was completely alert and furious. "I *told* you I didn't want that done," he growled.

"Mr. Zirkelbach, we thought you had encephalitis. You were incoherent."

"What do you mean by that?" he snapped.

"You couldn't answer questions."

"What questions?"

"Where you were. How old you are."

"Oh, those questions," Ralph scoffed. "I didn't answer

because they weren't important. You should have asked me about mathematical theories."

The doctor rolled her eyes.

Ralph continued. "You shouldn't have sent in some idiot to do the test."

The "idiot," the fellow who'd performed the spinal tap, turned scarlet. She scurried out of the room, and for the rest of Ralph's hospital stay we never saw her again. But her words during the procedure – "I can't get the needle in" – will echo in my mind forever.

"I'll order a consult with a neurosurgeon," Dr. Draper said in a tone of finality and left.

The door shut behind her, and the world turned black. I sat frozen by the bed, as helpless to move as Ralph. I stared at the place where his feet lay hidden beneath the sheet. Several years earlier I'd broken my foot. Struggling to get in and out of the car, navigate supermarket aisles, climb stairs, had taught me how vital locomotion is. But my broken bone had healed in a few weeks and I was back to normal. Would the hematoma do the same, or was it lodged forever in Ralph's spine?

My fault, my fault.

My signature set these events in motion.

I wanted to turn time back, grab the fellow's hand, stop the prick of the needle that had pierced Ralph's flesh. I wanted to go back to the day before that, erase the stroke of a pen, *my pen.*

The guilt still devils me. I was too quick to call the doctor, too trusting. I should have insisted that a neurologist do the spinal tap.

But time doesn't go backwards. Life doesn't hand out second chances. We live on, imprisoned by our mistakes.

◆◆◆

The next day we waited anxiously for the neurosurgeon. A robust, handsome man, he appeared after lunch, announced .that he had reviewed Ralph's files and had indeed identified a large hematoma pressing against the nerves. "Surgery to remove it would be dangerous," he said. "It could cause more bleeding, so we'll let it dissolve on its own."

"Will it?" I asked.

He assured us it would, but he couldn't say how long it would take. A couple of days, I told myself. A week at most.

Dr. Draper came in half an hour later. "You're going to be fine," she said confidently. "Those things always dissolve on their own." She left, not to return. Never, for the rest of Ralph's hospital stay, was she his attending physician.

Dr. Helm, Ralph's out-patient physician, was his next attending. I was glad to see her and welcomed her calm and pleasant attitude. But her news wasn't as promising as Dr. Draper's. It could be three or four months before the blood clot disappeared, she told us. Meanwhile, she scheduled Ralph for physical therapy. Left unsaid, was the phrase "just in case." Just in case, the hematoma didn't dissolve. Just in case.

Ralph, of course, was optimistic. After his first physical therapy session he told me he would be learning how to get about in a wheelchair for now. "And even if that's the best I can ever do, I'll manage."

His words encouraged me, but not enough. Guilt for signing the papers, remorse for my role in this horrible debacle plagued me. I'd been devastated over Ralph's leukemia. Now I'd be happy to settle just for that.

CHAPTER 17

As tension and guilt overwhelmed me, I began losing things. This was not new. Throughout my life, I frequently put things down and forgot where they were: a paper I needed, a book I was reading, my office key. On the day I defended my doctoral dissertation I misplaced the car keys and became near-hysterical before I found them.

Now that tendency became an over-riding pattern. I lost my wallet three times within a couple of weeks. Once I dropped it next to my car in my office parking lot, once I absentmindedly tossed it into the trash can in my office, another time I reached for my parking pass at the Medical Center and realized the wallet was missing. I turned around, made the twenty minute drive back to my office, and rushed into the building. In the middle of the afternoon I had gone downstairs to buy a Coke. I must have dropped the wallet by the vending machine, I thought. It wasn't there. I tried to get the man from the cleaning service to understand that it might be in the trash, but he didn't speak English and I don't speak Spanish. In tears I went into my office ... and found the wallet on the table next to the file cabinets.

In mid-May I attended the Houston Association for Communications Disorders' annual awards banquet. I didn't want to go, but I served as scholarship chair that year and part of my job was to hand out the checks to the scholarship recipients.

Although I enjoyed recognizing the winners, I felt removed from the cheerful throng, as if I were walking in my sleep. I barely responded to greetings from friends.

When I returned to the Cancer Institute, Ralph's room was empty. He'd been taken downstairs for an MRI. I sat down by the bed. I was tired and guilt-ridden, but more than that, I was angry. At fate, at the doctors, the hospital, the universe. Dammit, I wanted a vacation from this nightmare.

The phone rang. Lori wanted to know how Ralph was getting along. I began updating her.

The next thing I knew, someone called my name. I blinked at a worried looking nurse. "Mrs. Zirkelbach, are you all right?

Your daughter phoned and said you were talking to her and then you just stopped."

I'd fallen asleep. In the middle of a conversation.

"You need to see someone," Lori said. She meant a psychiatrist.

No, I thought. I would tough this out on my own. Friends complimented me on how strong I was. I liked that, and I agreed with them. Something inside me was growing, changing. For the first time in my life, I felt brave. Not quite brave enough to face the frightening future, but more capable of handling the present. Wouldn't getting help from a psychiatrist be weak?

But I knew I needed some time away from Ralph, who was becoming more and more difficult to deal with. As he lost control of his life – his ambulation, his bowels, his freedom – he became more controlling in the areas he could affect.

He refused to eat hospital food. He was unwilling to talk to the nutritionist but finally gave in. When she recommended certain soups, he insisted I call him from the grocery store so he could "supervise" my shopping for them. One day he asked me to exchange a can of soup for an identical one. I refused. "The store manager will think I'm nuts." And I began to wonder if Ralph was losing his mind.

Always a perfectionist about his files, he handed me papers to take home, insisting that checks be stapled to the left front of invoices, that they be filed precisely. One Sunday afternoon he gave me instructions by phone to straighten the files on his desk. "That goes on the right side in the second folder," he would say, or "Put the bill in the folder marked June and bring it to me along with the July folder."

"Okay."

"Are you sure you did it right way? Did you copy the check and staple it to the front?"

"Damn, no I didn't." I had never been involved in his business. Thank goodness for that, I thought. I didn't know if he behaved like this with his employees, but if so, I felt sorry for them.

"Can't you follow instructions?" he asked impatiently.

"Why do I have to copy all these checks anyway?" I protested. "Why don't you order checks with carbons?"

"Just keep going."

Halfway through the ordeal I began to cry. "I can't do this. I can never do it the way you want."

"What is your problem?" he growled

What was it? How hard could it be, and what a small thing he was asking. Still, I couldn't seem to please him and I hated myself, and him, in the process.

On a Sunday afternoon as I stood outside his room while the aide helped him bathe, I leaned against the door and shut my eyes. *"I've dreamed this,"* I told myself. *"When I open my eyes, I will wake up in my bed and all this will be just a nightmare."* Yes, the kind of vivid dream you remember with a pang throughout the day but that eventually fades away. I willed this to be true, but my wishes were the dream. Ralph and I had to live the reality.

One morning after I spent the night at the hospital, Ralph handed me a check to deposit at his bank. "Be sure to make a copy of the deposit slip," he ordered.

"No problem. I'll do that at my office and make the deposit on my way to lunch."

"No! I don't want it copied at your office. Copy it at home. Get it to the bank before two."

Dutifully, I did exactly as he insisted. I rushed home, copied the form, and raced to the bank. Would he have known the difference if I'd copied it on my office copier? Of course not, but apparently my obedience gene had kicked in.

Another day I came home from making a bank deposit and realized I didn't have the bank slip. I must have dropped it as I left the drive-in window. Panicked, I sped back to the bank, and ignoring the stares of other customers, crawled around the concrete parking lot until I found it.

I didn't understand Ralph's behavior; I understood mine even less.

Remembering the story told by the workshop presenter the previous fall about totaling her car in the aftermath of her grandchild's difficult birth, I feared I would wreck my car. I could hardly give up driving, but whenever I got behind the wheel, I was terrified.

I was losing my mind. Lori was right. I needed to see someone.

And so I began seeing Dr. Jessica Payne. She was someone to cry to, to vent to as I became more upset with the hospital and as I realized the tangled nature of Ralph's business affairs, which I'd never been aware of before. She assured me that taking Ambien nightly, which I'd been reluctant to do, would not be harmful. She encouraged me to spend fewer nights at the hospital and more at home. "You need the rest."

But I continued staying at the hospital at night. I would get up early, shower, eat breakfast, hurry home to feed our cats and be at work by 8:00. I saw clients until 6:30, and then rushed back to the hospital to eat a junk food dinner and spend the evening with Ralph.

During the night, I often woke to hear him talking with the aide who came to check his vital signs. "Are you okay?" I'd ask.

"Yeah. Go back to sleep."

I remembered a night years ago when we both awakened in the wee hours and couldn't fall back to sleep. "Let's go out for a midnight breakfast," I suggested.

We got up, dressed, and drove out of our neighborhood. No restaurants were open except IHOP, the International House of Pancakes. Better than nothing, we decided. I ordered blueberry pancakes; Ralph had a stack of silver dollar sized pancakes and an order of bacon. We laughed and talked as we ate. When we finished our breakfast, we drove home and went back to sleep. From then on IHOP became our "night place." On the few occasions we both woke up and couldn't sleep, we'd drive over and have pancakes. I wished we could do it again. I missed our freedom and our silliness. And our passion.

The romances I write are awash in passion: the adrenaline of sexual tension, the sweet rush of tenderness between two lovers; soulful glances, frantic couplings, explosive orgasms, warm afterglow. A romance novel is a happily-ever-after fantasy in which the reader imagines the hero and heroine's passion lasts forever and always at the same frenzied boiling point.

But we lived in the real world, not a fantasy. Passion was one part of our marriage but the rest was a balancing act between an outgoing computer geek and a shy language therapist, between a born procrastinator and an obsessive deadline-meeter, with love as a safety net. Love kept us going as we struggled from our very first days to build a marriage around a ready-made family. When we returned from the one-night "honeymoon" my housekeeper gave us as a wedding present, we found Bryan running a fever of 103 degrees. Welcome to the world of the Brady Bunch.

Our real marriage didn't end every day with a fade-out clinch. Some nights were hot and heavy; sometimes we were too tired for more than a goodnight mumble.

Real life marriage is disagreement and compromise and learning to let go of yesterday's annoyances. It's also laughter and discovery and quiet moments that need only the touch of one hand on another to know that two souls have become one.

Ralph and I shouted at each other, laughed together, sometimes misunderstood one another and other times communicated perfectly. We felt annoyed and tender and bored and surprised and renewed. Thirty-four years together, and I would give anything for a few more.

Despite his controlling behavior at that time, Ralph was pleased with his improvement. He could not yet stand by himself, but once helped to a wheelchair, could travel around the hospital on his own. This gave him the freedom to visit the cyber-center where he made copies and sent faxes. He could sit up in a chair and work on his computer, too, so all was right, or nearly right, with his world.

One afternoon I followed as he zoomed along the hallway in his wheelchair. Lori reported she'd accompanied him on a journey to the cafeteria, where she watched him down a greasy burger with gusto.

Dr. Helm said as soon as a room became available, he could transfer to the rehab floor, where he could get more intensive therapy.

Meanwhile, he told me the rehab doctor said he was an amazing patient, with his willingness to work hard and his positive attitude.

One troubling event occurred during those weeks. Ralph had a small wound on his lower back where the needle had penetrated during the lumbar puncture. Because it was located at a pressure point, the wound grew larger, deeper, and much more serious.

CHAPTER 18

On Monday, May 23, I celebrated my seventieth birthday. No, I didn't celebrate; I lived through it. Ordinarily, the beginning of a new decade would have been a cause for festivities and some angst at the idea of growing older; this year May 23 was merely a day, one with somewhat more significance than most, but on which I found it difficult to focus on anything beyond Ralph's illness, which permeated my life.

Lori took me to lunch to mark the occasion. We went to the Canyon Cafe, which featured southwestern food. We toasted my birthday with iced tea, and Lori gave me a jacket and a certificate for a massage.

After lunch I drove to my office and began my afternoon by looking for the folder of a child I'd evaluated for the Houston school district the Friday before. I had scored the test while waiting for an appointment with the doctor who, for the past year, had been following a nodule on my thyroid. Afterward, I returned to my office and, I was sure, brought the file with me.

It was nowhere to be found. I searched every place I could think of – the secretary's desk, the supply closet, the file cabinets. The folder wasn't there. I broke out in a sweat. In minutes my blouse was soaked, my hair plastered to my head. I called the doctor's office to see if I'd left the folder there; I checked the back seat and trunk of my car. No folder. Logically, I knew I could have the parent conference, and even write the report, without the folder. I easily recalled the test scores, but I wanted the hard copy. Tense and anxious, I saw my afternoon clients. Then I went home, and found the folder on the kitchen counter where I'd left it. Did Alzheimer's come on this suddenly or was I simply too stressed to think clearly?

Too worn out for a hospital visit, I went to bed. My seventieth birthday had been memorable, but not in the way I'd have chosen. On my sixtieth birthday Ralph and I went to hear the Houston Symphony play Beethoven's Ninth; we celebrated my sixty-fifth in Paris. We'd planned to go back this birthday, to wander the Louvre, hear a concert at Sainte Chapelle with late afternoon sunlight glowing through the stained glass windows, stroll along the Seine. Instead we faced the greatest challenge we could have imagined. And as I burrowed beneath the covers, I thought tearfully (and childishly) that on this milestone birthday I didn't even have a cake.

Dr. Payne suggested I begin a dose of Lexapro, an anti-depressant, anti-anxiety medication. Earlier I'd told myself to soldier on, but by now I was willing to try anything that would help me calm down. Within a few days of beginning the medication, I felt better, more in control. I firmly believe the medication made it possible for me to persevere through the worst months of my life. Contrary to what many think, I believe reliance on medication was not a weakness but a decision that enabled me to think clearly, to support my husband, and to stay healthy in the face of grief.

Ralph didn't take the jars of M&M's I'd set up to count his first hundred days to the hospital when he was readmitted, so at home I continued transferring candies from one jar to another as I counted down to Day One Hundred. One day I glanced at the remaining candies; there were too few. I counted. Only 16 were left, and there should have been more. Surely I hadn't begun losing M & M's. I guessed I had miscounted when I filled the first jar. Plenty of M&M's were left in the bag I'd bought. I added enough to jar number one to get the right amount.

Several days later more were missing. I counted and sure enough, the candies had decreased. Where could they have gone?

Suddenly I knew the answer. Allie, our housekeeper, had been snacking on them. I put a sign on the jar: *These candies are for counting, not eating.* The next time she came, Allie apologized profusely.

Near the end of May, Ralph moved downstairs to the fourth floor, to the rehab department. For me, this was an adjustment. Unlike the transplant floor, here the doors to patient's rooms could be open. Because Ralph's immune system was still weak,

I worried that germs might travel in from the hallway or other patient rooms, and I closed his door whenever I could.

There were fewer nurses on this floor, and each had more patients. And less patience. Used to immediate attention, Ralph did not get on well with the staff. He was demanding, controlling. He wanted his water glass put in a certain place on his bed tray, insisted on making the nurses or the therapy staff "wait a minute" until he finished whatever he was doing.

He became even more controlling with me. Each evening before I left, I had to put papers in one or another of the six file boxes he'd acquired, arrange mail he hadn't yet attended to in an order that made sense only to him. And, of course, he wanted the items on the bed tray put in order, too: the remote on the far left-hand corner, papers he was working on in the middle, the glass closest to the bed. I could go along with moving the glass; he had to be able to reach it. But the rest seemed unreasonable. And if I put anything an inch out of place, he fumed and submitted me to a lecture on my inability to follow directions.

I was glad to go home at night. On this floor, the lounge chair which unfolded into a bed was unwieldy and uncomfortable. My five foot one inch frame could barely fit into it. I wondered how an average-sized person could.

Meanwhile, Ralph's medical news was good. On Day Ninety post-transplant, he had a bone marrow aspiration with excellent results. The blood sample was clear of leukemia blasts and showed only female chromosomes, meaning his sister's blood had taken over and the transplant was successful.

We were thankful, but guilt still haunted me. If I hadn't signed the papers for the lumbar puncture, Ralph would be home now: moving, walking, enjoying a normal life.

The week after the bone marrow test Ralph developed an infection. He had to have a special diet while he took antibiotics. Unfortunately, nothing on this new diet appealed to him; everything was bland.

Ralph loved spicy food. He brought along a jar of hot sauce when we went on cruises and doctored his food if it wasn't hot enough to please him. Once we were downtown for some sort of festival and happened upon a chili tasting. "Yuck," I said.

"Come on," Ralph said. "If you go to this, I bet you'll get a book out of it."

Soon after the tasting I submitted a proposal to my editor for *The Great Chili Caper*, a detective spoof. To help with my research, Ralph joined the Houston chapter of the Chili Society and attended meetings faithfully, arriving home afterward reeking of cigarette smoke. For further research we drove to Terlingua, Texas for the International Chili Festival where we met chili aficionados from all over the country and tasted chili so hot it burned our guts, (One of the sponsors of the festival was Gaviscom, an antacid.) I persuaded a chili champion to let me include her recipe in my book.

No chili for Ralph now. But he was confident he'd lick the infection and be home by the end of June. He had someone come to our house and measure spaces for bars in the shower and by the toilet. He talked about ramps. On a Friday evening in early June he suggested we make a list of things to do to prepare for his homecoming.

As I got out a sheet of paper, the phone rang. His sister Sara was calling. I waited while they chatted and then said, "I'm going home. We'll make the list tomorrow."

I left the hospital, stopped at the garage entrance and glanced up at the stars. The June night was clear and a soft breeze brushed my cheek. I felt my tension drain away as I counted our blessings. The transplant was a success, Ralph would come home soon, and surely, back in his own world, his good nature would return .

CHAPTER 19

At home I went into my study and opened the file I was working on, a chapter midway through my Silhouette book. My deadline was September 15, and despite the chaos around me, I was progressing on schedule.

While I was typing, the phone rang. My daughter-in-law Monica's name popped up on Caller ID. Probably wanted to know if I could babysit the next evening.

"Um, Michael didn't want me to call you, but I thought I should. He's in the hospital."

"Wh...why?"

"Just for observation. He's had chest pains."

I couldn't get enough breath to answer. Michael had had a serious heart attack seven years earlier, at age thirty-four. Not another one. Not again, and especially not now.

I finally managed to ask, "What happened? Where is he?"

"In short-term care at the McKenzie Heart Center. It's not a heart attack, but they're keeping him overnight."

I broke into a cold sweat. It started at the top of my head and within seconds my hair was drenched. A few seconds more and my t-shirt was soaked. "I, um, don't think I can drive," I said. I glanced at my shaking hands and knew without a doubt if I got behind the wheel, I would crash my car.

"You don't need to come. I'll call you back as soon as I know something." She hung up.

Automatically, I saved my file and turned off the computer before I slid to the floor and curled up in a ball. Though covered with sweat, I shivered. Time seemed to stop and then spin crazily back and forth.

Seven years earlier I got the call from Monica on a January night as I was getting ready for bed: "I think Michael's having a heart attack."

I ran outside to Ralph's office in what had once been our garage and told him what had happened. "We have to go to the hospital." Michael and Monica, married only a few months, lived north of Houston, in Tomball, near Compaq Computers, where Michael worked. Tomball was an hour's drive from our house. All the way there, I remembered my former mother-in-law telling me how she rushed to the hospital when her oldest son had a heart attack, asked where his room was, and was told in a bored voice, "Oh, he died." I pictured that happening to me.

On the way I asked Ralph to call Ginny, our office manager, and have her cancel an early conference the next morning. I couldn't remember her phone number; I couldn't recall where I kept it. Instead, he called my partner, woke her, and gave her the news.

At the hospital I found Michael shaky but alert. Weak with relief, I clutched his hand.

Two days later he was transferred to the McKenzie Heart Center for an angiogram, but we assumed he'd be discharged the next day, so I went to my office for my afternoon appointments. Lori reached me there. "Michael's having a triple bypass in the morning."

I stumbled into the office waiting room, and Kelli Graham, whose child was next, noticed my pale face and asked what was wrong. "Give me the phone numbers," she said. "and I'll cancel the rest of your appointments. Go be with your son." I've never forgotten Kelli's kindness.

Because he and Monica had sold their house just two weeks before, Michael was discharged to my house after his surgery. They and Marco lived with us for two years while they built a new house and had a baby. Gabriella spent her first year in our home, and I believe that's why we have a special bond.

Ralph was with me that time, but now I was on my own. When I could move, I crawled to the bedroom. I don't know why I left my study with the phone next to my computer; the bedroom seemed safer, I suppose. I sat on the floor and called Ralph's room. The line was busy. He was still talking to his sister. I dialed Lori's number. No answer. No answer on her cell phone either. She had to be out somewhere on the singles' scene, where I couldn't contact her.

Ralph's line remained busy. Fingers shaking, I called the nursing station on his floor. "I need to talk to Mr. Zirkelbach right away," I told the man who answered.

He came back in a few minutes. "He's on the phone. He said he'll be off in just a minute."

I knew Ralph's "just-a-minute" line only too well. "Tell him to get off *now*," I shouted into the phone. "It's an emergency."

Finally, finally he answered my call.

I began to cry. "Michael ..."

"What's wrong?" Ralph said. "Tell me what happened." This was the take-charge Ralph I knew, competent but soothing at the same time. This was exactly what I needed.

Between gasps, I told him. "I don't know what to do. I don't even know exactly where Michael is," I sobbed.

"Don't try to drive," he said. "I'll call someone to stay with you."

"Call Marla."

While I waited for Ralph to call back, I sat on the floor with my head in my hands. *I should be hurting*, I thought. *Why am I not hurting?* I couldn't feel anything but sweat.

Seven years ago I'd felt as if I were sliding into a hole – a deep, dark well; this time I sensed a whirlpool tossing me round and round. I couldn't hang onto anything. I couldn't think. What if I had to go to the hospital? Where was Lori? What if Ralph couldn't reach Marla? How would I manage alone all night when I couldn't even get myself up from the floor?

The phone rang, loud as a siren. Was it Monica? With life going the way it had the last few weeks she could only have bad news. I reached for the phone; it fell out of my hand and bounced on the floor.

I grabbed it and put it to my ear without looking at the Caller ID. *Please be Monica. Please let her say it's a mistake.* "Hello."

It was Ralph. "Marla's on her way. I'm trying to get hold of Lori."

Again, his voice calmed me. Even though we weren't together, even though he could do nothing but make phone calls, I felt better listening to him talk. My tears dried.

A few minutes later the doorbell rang and Marla, her pajamas tossed in a bag, stepped inside. I began to cry again. Marla sat with me in the living room while I held the phone, waiting for it to ring.

Lori called first. The man she was dating had come to town,

they'd gone out for a hamburger, and she'd left her cell phone at home. I gave her the news, and she promised to be at the hospital the next day.

Then Monica called. Michael was all right, but he was frightened. So was she; so was I. I told her I'd see Michael the next morning. Hopefully, by then I'd be able to drive.

I said good night to Marla and we both went to bed. Toby, my cat, curled up against me as if he knew I needed the warmth of his little body.

I've studied theories of non-verbal communication, but that night they became reality. Skin is our oldest, largest sense organ. Touch has a deeper meaning than speech; it bypasses the thinking part of our brain and reaches our emotional core. Without Ralph's touch but reassured by Toby's nearness, I fell asleep with the sound of my pet's gentle purr in my ears.

Early the next morning I drove to the Heart Center. I found Michael, weak and pale, in a glassed-in room a few steps from a nurses' station. The pains of the day before were a precursor. Earlier this morning he felt the crushing pain of a full-blown heart attack. Now we waited for his cardiologist.

The doctor confirmed what had happened. Arteries were clogged again, only seven years after his original attack. This was genetic, the cardiologist said, verifying what we already knew, that Michael had inherited a predisposition for coronary disease from his father. Another bypass was scheduled for Monday.

We sat silently, listening to the report. I didn't want to be quiet. I wanted to scream at the unfairness of this. To my son, to his family, to me. Another emotion to master, another sob to stifle. I would not cry in front of Michael. I needed to be calm, just as I was for Ralph.

We turned on the television and watched the Home Channel. Michael and Monica were remodeling their house. The program kept Michael's mind on that instead of on the impending surgery and the affect his illness might have on his family, especially Gabriella.

On the remodeling show, a professional football player planned a home makeover to surprise his wife, who was away on a business trip. We saw the changes in decor and the wife's surprise when she opened the front door. Funny how vividly I recall that show, even the wife's exclamation of delight when she saw her newly decorated living room.

During Michael's surgery seven years earlier, I watched the Jerry Springer show for my one and only time. I remember the book I read when the TV show ended: *The Fifties* by David Halberstam.

Details always stick in your mind after a crisis: the dress you wore when you got bad news, the meal you ate just before a disaster, the TV show you watched to keep from fearing that your son would die at thirty-four, or now at forty-one.

Early in the afternoon I left Michael's room to visit Ralph. The Heart Center and the Cancer Institute shared entrances into my familiar stomping ground, Garage 2. Although it was still early June, summer was firmly entrenched along the Texas Gulf Coast. The afternoon was hot and humid, and the garage was stifling. The smell of exhaust, the sunlight shining through the openings and bouncing off hoods of cars made me dizzy as I walked from the one hospital to the other.

Outside the garage door a Cancer Institute patient stood smoking, seeming unaware of the irony of a cancer victim dragging an IV pole and puffing on a cigarette. Afraid the stench of smoke would make me nauseous, I held my breath as I passed him, then hurried across the street and up to Ralph's room.

I stepped inside and began to cry. He patted the bed, and I sat down beside him, laid my head on his chest and sobbed out all the morning's grief.

He stroked my hair. "Michael will be all right," he murmured. "I wish I could take care of you."

"You are, right now," I sniffled. His tender touch on my hair reassured me, made me believe all would be well.

After a while, I curled up in a chair, shut my eyes, and listened as the occupational therapist worked with Ralph. He told her about our trip to Antarctica and how much fun we'd had.

What if we'd waited to go? as Ralph had suggested. "We'll go next year ... the year after." Then he wouldn't have those memories to cherish. I wished I could run the clock back three years and live that adventure again.

◆◆◆

I spent Sunday night in Ralph's room, got up at 5:00 a.m., ate breakfast, of course, and walked over to the Heart Center. Michael's surgery was scheduled for 7:00 but it was postponed until 8:00. Another hour of anxiety.

All I could think when the orderlies finally arrived to take Michael to surgery was *Please let him be all right.* What I said to him though was, "We'll be here. You'll be fine, and remember, you're not living at my house another two years."

We went downstairs to the waiting room for cardiac patients. Near the elevators we saw a large family literally camping out, with sleeping bags, blankets, coolers, and other necessities. Inside, the waiting room was already crowded at 8:00 a.m. By now, I was used to this scene. A different hospital, a different illness, but the same anxious faces, strained postures; the same hands holding unread magazines, half-empty coffee cups. Faces showing the same mingled emotions of hope and despair.

Lori, Monica, and I sat and waited. No minutes crawl by as slowly as those spent waiting for a loved one in surgery, especially when that loved one is your child. Children are supposed to do the waiting, parents to be the patients.

I thought of mothers with offspring in the armed forces, serving in Iraq or Afghanistan. How did they fall asleep at night? How did they keep their lives going – eating breakfast, folding laundry, shopping for groceries – knowing their sons or daughters could be killed or maimed at any moment? I had to wait only a few hours to know Michael's outcome and I was sick with fear. Knowing Ralph could be taken from me was heartbreaking, but the fear of losing the son I'd nourished in my womb, brought into the world and watched grow from infancy to manhood was unbearable.

I pictured Michael at the beginning of his life, a placid, chubby infant. (He weighed nearly ten pounds at birth.) After an initial bout of jealousy, Lori was entranced by her little brother. My parents came for a visit when he was a month old, and Lori grabbed their arms and pulled them into his room. "Grandma, Grandpa, this is Michael. He makes pee pee up in the air."

Michael's placidity vanished with his infancy. He was an active, mischievous preschooler who got into everything. Eventually we put hooks under our kitchen cabinet doors and fastened rubber bands from the hooks to the cabinet knobs so he wouldn't open them when he climbed up on the counter.

His favorite toy was a terry cloth dog called Elmer. Michael sucked his thumb and rubbed Elmer against his cheek, until one day the toy mysteriously vanished. Years later I found a mangled Elmer under a shrub where Lori admitted she'd hidden him. I ran him through the washer and still have him in my closet along with other mementos of my son and daughter's childhoods.

By the time he was a teenager and "Beau" of a girl's club, Michael had developed a sense of humor honed by "Monty Python" and "Saturday Night Live." He and a couple of his buddies made funny movies, one of them a take-off on PI shows. He left for college, but came home often during his first year, lugging his dirty laundry. After graduate school he lived in New York for a couple of years and I had the chance to realize a fantasy I'd had since his childhood: to spend a night at his apartment and leave a mess in *his* kitchen after the next morning's breakfast.

Losing him wasn't possible. I wouldn't let myself think it.

Monica's sister arrived, and she, Lori and Monica chatted. Their voices grated on my ears. I couldn't join in the talk. I concentrated on breathing.

Finally we got the report that Michael was out of surgery. He'd had some breathing problems but otherwise was doing well. Monica and I went into the Cardiac Care Unit (CCU) to take a quick look at him. He was asleep, hooked up to a monitor, a breathing tube in place.

I remembered his last cardiac surgery. I visited one morning while the ventilating tube was still in. He motioned for a paper and pencil and wrote me a note: "This nurse is a bitch." Before I could crumple the paper, the nurse glanced over my shoulder and read it. Fortunately, today's nurse seemed pleasant. "We'll take good care of him," she promised.

Lori, Monica, her sister and I went to lunch at the Commons, a garage-restaurant area a block's walk from The Heart Center.

As we headed over, my hip began to hurt. I'd been diagnosed with a degenerative disc, which flared up every now and then. Why did it have to do so now, at the worst possible time? I could hardly walk, and I certainly couldn't keep up with these young women who exercised daily. Every few feet I had to stop until the pain went away. But despite that, I felt more hopeful. The worst was over for Michael.

I spent the next few days traveling back and forth between hospitals. Michael was still on a ventilator. Whenever they woke him, he fought the tube and they couldn't remove it, so he was given a morphine drip to keep him relaxed. Each time I came, it was the same story. I began to fear he'd not be able to come off the tube, but finally they were able to take it out. The next time we visited, Michael said in a raspy voice, "Everyone around here is wearing masks."

"They're supposed to be. You're in a hospital."

◆◆◆

Meanwhile, at the Cancer Institute Ralph's doctors voiced concern about the pressure sore that had developed from the prick during the lumbar puncture. The wound had not healed; they said it was large and infected. I heard this but didn't really process it. I was too overcome with all that was happening.

Michael, Ralph. Heart disease, cancer. Hospital, work. I was overwhelmed. I wonder now how I kept going; yet I did. The whirlpool didn't suck me down. I fought it and refused to let it get the best of me. Like the romance heroines of today who no longer depend on the hero to ride to their rescue, I saved myself.

CHAPTER 20

Friday, June 10, Day 100, was almost here. With Ralph's bone marrow now clear of blasts, it should have been a day of celebration.

But Thursday morning I got a phone call from a nurse on the rehab floor. Her accent was foreign. Filipino? Japanese? "The doctor scheduled a meeting at 1:00 this afternoon. You must be there."

"What's the meeting about?"

"I can't say," she answered.

Alarmed, I asked, "Why?"

"I can't say."

What secret were they keeping? Was Ralph dying? "Can I bring my daughter?"

"Maybe."

By now I was frantic. "Find out."

"I call you back."

"No. I'll hold on."

In a moment another voice came on. "This is Donna Olson, the nurse practitioner. Can I help you?"

"You can tell me what's going on."

"It's just a care meeting. 1:00."

"I want my daughter to come."

"Of course."

"This is a terrible time for me. My son just had heart surgery."

"I heard," Donna said. "I'm sorry. Is he all right?"

"He's doing fine, but I'm upset."

"No reason to be upset about the meeting." I didn't believe that for an instant. "We'll see you at 1:00."

"Can Ralph be at the meeting, since it's about him?"

"Um, okay."

I hung up and called Lori. Yes, she'd be there. What did I do next? Ate lunch, of course. I gave myself plenty of time to find a parking space in the garage and walk to Ralph's room. Soon after I got there, Dr. Helm rushed in. She had just learned about the meeting, so she couldn't enlighten me on what was going to happen.

She turned to Ralph. "Mr. Zirkelbach, they tell me you aren't eating. You're off the fresh fruit and vegetable restriction. How about some fruit? Would you like that?"

"Watermelon," Ralph said.

"I'll see that you get it."

Lori arrived a little before 1:00. I went to the nurses' station to let them know we were ready. But "they," whoever they were, were not.

We waited nervously. Why the delay? Why the secrecy? Or perhaps there wasn't a secret; perhaps the nurse, not fluent in English, hadn't meant she couldn't tell, but that she didn't know what we were meeting about.

Finally at 3:30 the door opened. Ralph's current doctor, a dapper man named Dr. Chan, came in followed by Donna, the rehab physician, a dark-haired woman from the patient advocacy office, and a nurse. Dr. Chan began. "Mr. Zirkelbach, you have not been cooperating with the rehab therapists."

Ralph started to respond, but the rehab doctor cut in. "To be on this floor, you have to be involved in therapy six hours a day. You have not." This impatient, irritated doctor was the man who'd once said Ralph was the most motivated patient he'd ever had.

"We know you have an infection," Dr. Chan continued, "and the rehab people have made allowances for that."

The rehab doctor went on. "Every time one of the therapists comes in, you ask them to wait. You say you're busy, to come back later."

The doctors gave Ralph no chance to reply. They kept talking, their voices harsh, their words flying at him like bullets. They stood in a circle around the bed, like bullies surrounding a defenseless kid on the playground.

"They have other patients to see," the rehab doctor said. "If you tell them to come back later or to wait, then you don't get your therapy because they have to work with other people."

"And your wound," Dr. Chan continued. "It's not healing because you're leaning against it all the time when you're up in your chair. The therapist has asked you to sit leaning forward, but you don't listen."

I glanced at Lori, and she nodded. Because she came during the day, she'd seen this happen.

"You can't stay on this floor," the rehab doctor said. "We're sending you back to the transplant floor. The plastic surgeon will work on your wound, and we'll give you a therapy schedule. You'll have to meet it."

Ralph tried to speak, tried to say *they* were responsible for the wound, for the paralysis, but he couldn't get the words out. All he managed was an incoherent mumble.

Why didn't I jump in to defend him? I hated the way they spoke to Ralph, but I, too, had seen his oppositional behavior the past few weeks.

"We'll move you tomorrow," Dr. Chan said, and they trooped out.

Lori and I sat in silence. Ralph shut his eyes and went to sleep.

I went home angry at Ralph for his "wait-a-minute" attitude, which I completely believed was true. A couple of years ago we had taken a Spanish course as a prelude to a trip to Spain to immerse ourselves in the language. That course almost killed our marriage by requiring far more time than we expected. Every evening I sat down in the living room with the course video ready to go, and Ralph would say, "I'll be with you in a few minutes." The minutes always stretched to several hours, and it was well past 10:00 before he started. He was "too busy" to take the required tests. And *he* was the one who was so eager to learn Spanish. I finished the course; he didn't. By the end, we were barely speaking to each other

So I empathized with the therapists assigned to work with him. I knew exactly how exasperating he could be.

On the other hand, I was furious at Dr. Chan. I didn't like his arrogant manner, his implication that the infected wound was Ralph's fault, that the hospital and their treatment weren't amiss. Easy to tell someone, "You're a bad patient. That's why you're not improving." Easy and unfair.

Instead of the uplifting, cheerful book I'd planned to write about Ralph's illness, I decided I'd write one exposing the dark side of medicine: heartless doctors, rushed and overworked staff, hospital mishaps. No matter how reputable the medical establishment, no matter how cutting-edge the treatment, things go wrong. And the blame is often laid at the patient's feet.

The next morning I dropped the last M&M into the hundred day jar and stared at the now full container. This wasn't the hundredth day I'd pictured. I picked up the jars and put them out of sight, in a cabinet where they still sit today.

The phone rang when I was getting ready to leave for the hospital. "We have a room upstairs for your husband. We'll move him this afternoon. You can take his office supplies home."

Six heavy boxes? "I can't carry them. I have a bad back," I said.

"Transportation will take them to the car for you."

"Yeah," I said, "and who will take them out of the car when I get home? Besides, my husband will need them. Transportation can move them upstairs when he goes."

The nurse muttered something I couldn't hear and hung up.

When I arrived at the hospital, I found Ralph asleep. I tried to wake him. "They're moving you upstairs today, remember?"

"No."

"You'll be back on the eleventh floor."

"No."

That was his reply, no matter what I said.

Upstairs, he was equally unresponsive.

The only room available on the transplant floor had a special oxygen filtering system for severely immuno-suppressed patients. A glass-paned door led to a small entranceway and another similar door opened into the room. This made the space smaller than most, which meant that Ralph's many file boxes, which Transportation had shoved against a wall, left me little room to move. Closet space was at a minimum. I stuffed in what I could and sat down amidst the clutter. The tiny room made me feel as if I were being choked.

Ralph lay in the bed, his eyes shut. I tried calling to him, nudging him, but he only grunted. He never opened his eyes.

When the nurse, whom I knew and liked, came in, I told her about Ralph's unresponsiveness, which was similar to his behavior before the fateful lumbar puncture. She called Dr. Chan.

As much as I disliked this doctor, I was glad he did not

treat this as an emergency. He told me he would ask both a neurologist and a psychiatrist to evaluate Ralph. Meanwhile, we would wait. If Dr. Draper had waited when this happened before, Ralph might have been home with me, celebrating one hundred days free of leukemia.

And yet ...

Was waiting really a good idea? Would Ralph get worse if nothing was done? And what *could* be done?

The nurse appeared again and said the doctor had ordered a sitter to stay with Ralph during the night. I went downstairs to eat and when I returned, the sitter was in the room. A tall, African-American man who was not particularly reassuring, he had appropriated the room's only comfortable chair and made no move to vacate it for me. I sat in an upright, wooden chair, and the sitter and I watched the NBA finals.

How could I concentrate on basketball? As always, sports kept my mind off the horror of reality. After the game I went home.

The neurologist came the next morning. He said Ralph's condition could be a result of medication, infection, or chance. We would continue to wait.

In the afternoon the psychiatrist, a large, Nordic looking woman with an accent to match, arrived. She sat beside the bed. "Mr. Zirkelbach, I'm Dr. Weller. Would you like to talk to me?"

"No."

"Are you depressed?"

"No."

"Angry?"

"No ... I don't know."

She said she'd order Haldol, a strong, anti-psychotic drug, and she'd be back Monday.

The evening was a repeat of the preceding one. Ralph didn't seem to be getting better, but he wasn't worse either. Exhausted, I left.

The next morning the phone woke me. "Hi," Ralph said. "Are you up?"

"Ralph?" He sounded so normal, I thought I was still asleep and had dreamed him.

"Yeah, have you had breakfast yet? Are you coming today?"

"I'll be there in an hour."

When I arrived, he was awake and hungry. "Call Room Service," he said, "and order a peach smoothie."

"They don't make peach." I knew the smoothie menu by heart.

"Ask them anyway."

"But ..."

"Ask."

The nurse who was in the room winked at me. "Mr. Zirkelbach is back."

And so he was. Whatever caused the lapse was over. And I wished I could press a Rewind button and go back to the episode in April, have Dr. Draper call a neurologist or just wait for Ralph to get better on his own.

Meanwhile, I continued my walks back and forth between the Cancer Institute and the Heart Center. Michael was recovering quickly, and on Father's Day he got permission for Gabriella to visit him. She brought such joy to her father, and watching them walk along the hall hand in hand touched me deeply.

◆◆◆

Within a few days Ralph moved down the hall to a regular sized room where he and I could spread out. There were large windows looking west and the room was filled with light. He asked if I intended to spend the night, but Dr. Payne had firmly insisted I sleep at home, so I said no. But I told him that every morning when I woke, I imagined he was beside me.

"That's nice," he said, smiling.

As lonely as it was, I soon realized I preferred being at home. Within a few days, Ralph plummeted into a severe depression and nothing pleased him.

A plastic surgeon had worked on the wound and Ralph was required to turn every two hours and to stay off his back while healing from the procedure. This meant he could not use his computer. Or at least he couldn't use it the way he liked. Michael stated he often worked on his laptop while lying in bed on his side, but Ralph refused to even consider this. It was his way or no way, and clearly "his way" was out of the question.

The nutritionist measured his food consumption. It was practically nil. He could eat anything he wanted now, but he seemed to be deliberately starving himself.

I asked why he didn't watch TV, since he had always kept a TV playing on his desk at home while he worked. He said it bothered his eyes. He didn't want to read either and barely scanned the newspaper.

I offered to bring my tape recorder so he could listen to some of the courses I had bought from The Teaching Company. He agreed and insisted I buy a new tape recorder, so to placate him, I did. He listened to part of one tape. "Never mind," he muttered and returned the rest of the courses to me.

My spirits fell along with Ralph's. Now it was full summer and the sunlight in his hospital room seemed harsh. At night the dark was stark and unfriendly.

When I visited, Ralph barely spoke except to complain that the therapy team had not figured out a way for him to use his computer.

One afternoon as I was unhappily driving back to my office, my cell phone rang. The social worker from the transplant floor was calling. "Your husband says he needs to use his computer."

"Yes, are you working out an arrangement for him?"

"No, ma'am," he said. "I'm just calling to find out if he needs the computer."

"Didn't *he* tell you that?"

"Yes."

"Then why are you asking me?" I said, annoyed. "Okay, I'm verifying that he needs it."

"Ah," he said in a sad voice, "that's a problem."

"Can you work out a way for him to use it? A special chair or something?"

"That's not my job."

"What *is* your job?" I inquired. "A couple of months ago I called about getting transportation, and you said, 'That's a problem,' but you didn't help me or even try. Now you're calling me about the computer and when I ask you to do something, you say, 'That's a problem.' Is that your job, to say,

'That's a problem'?"

"Yes, ma'am, my job is to verify that there is a problem."

"But not to do anything to fix it, huh?" By now I was shouting. "Don't call me again. Ever. Got it?"

"Yes, ma'am."

He never called again.

I had to tell Ralph he wouldn't get his computer back.

I think that was when he decided to die.

CHAPTER 21

Ralph had always been fascinated with technology. The loss of his computer, even temporarily, cut him to the quick. His ego and his identity as a professional and as a businessman, were tied to that machine.

Now this man, who prided himself on his logical approach to the world, became irrational. He proposed installing a computer in the ceiling or finding a chair that he could sit in sideways, and when Lori or I argued that such things made no sense, he accused us of not being on "his side." The suggestion that he would get his computer back eventually when his wound healed did not improve his outlook. He wanted it *immediately*. And he couldn't have it.

One evening after work I entered Ralph's room to find his friend Darlene packing boxes. Darlene was an accountant with a smoke-roughened voice and gray hair pulled up in a top knot that gave her head the look of a decaying pineapple. We greeted each other, but Ralph did not say why she was there. He simply continued giving her instructions. I was embarrassed to ask in front of her what was going on.

When she left, I scowled at him. "What was that about?"

"She's going to take care of my clients."

That was the worst decision Ralph ever made.

♦♦♦

His attitude continued to deteriorate. He began having panic attacks, feeling as if he couldn't breathe. The psychiatrist kept him on Haldol, and the psychiatric social worker visited him. Months later when I read her notes in his medical records, I saw the comment: "The patient was not pleasant." Well, no, but he'd lost everything that mattered in life. Who would be?

Life spun out of control for both of us. The nurse suggested Ralph have a sitter again at night. That was a good idea, I thought. No longer could I spend any nights at the hospital; I was too tired. Most days I longed for the oblivion of sleep and counted the hours until I could swallow an Ambien, get into bed and blot out all the worries of the day.

One morning Ralph confided to me that his current sitter told him the Franklin Cancer Institute was not a good place for orthopedic rehabilitation. "She's planning to open a convalescent home for rehab patients ... as soon as she has $20,000."

"Oh, my God. You didn't offer to lend her money, did you?" My over-generous husband would be just the one to do that, or even to give it to her gratis. *Please, not this,* I thought. *Especially not now.* We were approaching the limit of Ralph's Medicare coverage. If Ralph didn't get out of the hospital soon, we'd be in desperate straits.

"I didn't give her any money," Ralph said, "but I want you to call her."

"Why? Is she certified in some kind of therapy? Can she give IV's?"

"No."

"What kind of place can she open for $20,000? Think about it."

"Just call her," he insisted.

This time, I didn't follow orders.

I had one thing to be cheerful about. Michael was home and doing well. He and Monica decided to have a smaller version of their usual Fourth of July celebration. They lived near downtown so after dinner everyone walked a couple of blocks to the best site for viewing the annual fireworks display.

Last year I'd brought an Independence Day pie. I'd found the recipe in a magazine in my office waiting room. The pie contained layers of strawberry jello, Kool Whip, and blueberry jello on a graham cracker crust. Red, white, and blue. Unfortunately, the yellowish graham crackers turned the blueberry jello green so the pie wasn't exactly what I intended. This year I tried again and managed to keep the two layers separate so the colors were right. But on Monday, July 4, I was too overwrought and exhausted to go to the party. I curled up in bed and watched the fireworks on TV. During the next couple of days, ravenous for sugar, I devoured the whole pie myself.

◆◆◆

On July 5, I got up early and was about to get into the shower when Ralph called. "Get down here," he said. "I fell out of bed."

"Are you hurt?"

"No, but come on."

For the first and probably only time in my life, I skipped breakfast. Grabbing some clothes, I sped to the hospital.

Ralph looked the same – no bruises I could discern, but he was distraught. "I reached for my water glass at night. They put it too far away, so I lost my balance."

"How did you get up?" I asked, imagining him lying on the floor for hours before someone found him.

"I yelled and they came."

I strode outside to the nursing station. "What happened last night?" I demanded.

"He was part way out of bed, but the rails stopped his fall," the nurse replied.

"He's upset." So was I.

We had a new doctor this week, Dr. DeMarco, who would become my favorite. Approachable, kind, humorous and optimistic, he was popular with patients and staff alike. He assured me Ralph was unharmed, and then made a suggestion. "Mr. Z, you've been stuck in your bed for some weeks now. Would you like to go out in the wheelchair for an hour a day?"

Ralph's eyes filled with tears as he nodded.

"We'll get you started as soon as possible."

When the doctor left, Ralph was so excited, he could barely speak. Maybe, I thought, this was what he needed to help him recover his optimism and the will to overcome his illness. Exhausted from stress but encouraged, I left the hospital and went to an appointment with my new allergist. The previous one, whom I really liked, had moved away.

I liked this man, too. But when I told him my allergies weren't bothering me much, he said, "That happens as you get older and your immune system changes, but now you're more likely to get cancer."

Thanks a lot, doc. Just what I wanted to hear this morning.

At work after my doctor's appointment I took out a set of

miniature plastic doll furniture, a mother doll and a baby doll out of my bag and set them up on the table. Two-year-old Lisa and I took the dolls through their day.

"Mommy says, 'Time to get up. Are you hungry, baby?'"

"Baby hungwy," Lisa answered.

"What do you want?"

"Baby want tewul."

"Cereal, mmm. Sit down, baby. Mommy will get it."

"Baby eat it a' up."

"Mommy says, 'Let's watch TV.'"

"Okay. Baby si' couch."

"Click." I pretended to turn on the TV.

"No, no," Lisa said. "Mo'."

"Mo," I muttered. I didn't have a piece of furniture that sounded like "mo." Usually I could figure out what children meant. Maybe "mo" meant "more." "More cereal first?" I asked.

"No, mo'."

Mo...stro. "Does she want to go out in the stroller?"

Lisa gave me a disgusted look and pointed again to the tiny TV. "Mo," she demanded. "Mo...t."

Ah. I translated, "Remote."

"Uh huh."

Whoops. The set was out of date. "Sorry, no remote," I said. "It's lost. We'll just turn the TV on. See. Click."

How wonderful it was to be able to laugh at something.

The next day Ralph grumbled, "Dammit, they said the wheelchair's not ready yet. Do you think they're putting me off?"

"I'm sure if Dr. DeMarco promised you a wheelchair, there'll be one," I assured him. I went to the nurses' desk to remind them he was waiting anxiously for the chair.

I felt uncharacteristically optimistic. Once he could get out of bed, even for a short time, I hoped Ralph would recover his interest in the outside world. Maybe he'd start watching television again or reading the newspaper.

No longer a news junkie, the following day he was unaware that bombs were detonated in the London subway and fifty-two people were dead. Ordinary people going to ordinary places suddenly and unwittingly became a part of history. How senseless and sad.

I mentioned this news to Ralph, but in a measure of his apathy, he made no comment. Instead he grumbled that items on his bed tray were out of place. I went home feeling frustrated.

Friday I was still tired and stressed, and I didn't want to go to the hospital. I called the psychiatric social worker to get her view on Ralph's anxiety attacks and difficult behavior. She told me what I'd heard before, that he was battling for control.

After our conversation, I felt guilty. How could I be angry with Ralph when so much had been taken from him? Couldn't I be a more understanding wife? A better person? I'd go to the hospital after all.

When I got to the eleventh floor around 4:00, I could see that Ralph's door was open, which meant he wasn't in the room. "I guess he's finally out in the wheelchair," I said and waved at the current fellow as I strolled past the nursing station.

The fellow came around the desk and waylaid me before I reached the room. "Mrs. Zirkelbach, I just called you at home. We'd like to talk to you."

I stopped. "Okay."

"This way." He led me toward a small conference room and motioned to a chair. Three more people crowded in with us: the head nurse and two others, their faces solemn.

What was going on? Had Ralph done something tacky and they'd decided to kick him out of the hospital? Or worse, had he signed himself out?

"Mrs. Zirkelbach," the charge nurse said, "your husband had a little accident."

What did "little" mean? "What happened?" I asked.

"He, ah … we believe he fell out of the wheelchair."

The floor seemed to drop out from under me, but my voice sounded perfectly normal when I asked, "Wasn't he belted in?"

"No."

"What happened?"

"Well, we don't know exactly, but he was outside with the occupational therapist and he hit his head. They took him to the emergency room to take care of it."

I stood on wobbly legs. "I'll go down. I know where the ER is."

"They're going to do a C-T scan, just as a precaution, so he may be in radiology. Why don't you wait in his room?"

"All right." I went back to his room, turned on CNN, and watched the latest news from London.

The minutes passed slowly, but I wasn't too worried. Ralph had probably been shaken up a bit, and checking him over was the sensible thing to do when his blood counts were still dangerously low. I didn't think to wonder why it had taken four people to give me the news of his accident. Around 5:00 the charge nurse came in. "There's a problem. Mr. Zirkelbach is in Intensive Care."

Addled, I stared at her. "I don't know where that is."

"Downstairs, on the seventh floor. Come on, I'll go with you."

Downstairs. I'd heard *that* word before. The Ledermans. Sylvia had gone "downstairs." Was it a stop on the way to the morgue?

CHAPTER 22

The charge nurse and two other nurses herded me into an elevator. Why were there so many of them? The four of us stood silently. The elevator seemed to barely move. I wanted to get downstairs in a hurry; I didn't want to get there at all and face what was coming.

Why didn't one of the nurses say something? What was it they weren't telling me?

Finally I blurted, "Is ... he ... dead?"

"No, no," they chorused. "He was asking for you. They're stitching him up."

Why in Intensive Care? I wondered but I couldn't get the words out.

The elevator opened. I'm sure the seventh floor was like all the others I'd visited, but it looked ... grim. Everything was white – walls, doors, floors – but a dull white that didn't seem to reflect any light.

It was hard to walk, even harder to breathe, but I followed the nurses step by step through a maze of corridors. I felt as if we were walking through a dungeon. Maybe they'd lied to me. Maybe this *was* the way to the morgue.

We reached an area of small rooms with sliding glass doors that looked out on a nursing station. Two of the nurses stopped, and the charge nurse led me to one of the cubicles and then stood back, and I saw my husband.

Surrounded by doctors and nurses, he was propped up on the bed. He looked like a character in a horror movie, his left temple bruised and bloody against the pasty white of his face. His eyes were wild, and a horrible gurgling sound came from his chest. He stretched out his hand when he saw me, and I went to him and took it.

"I ... hit ... head," he whispered, and I felt the last vestiges of our life shatter around us.

"Mrs. Zirkelbach, you need to leave now so we can work on him," one of the doctors told me.

"I'll be back," I promised Ralph and backed out of the room.

Another doctor followed me. "He's bleeding down his trachea," he informed me. "We need to put in a breathing tube."

This was a decision I'd never dreamed of having to make. Were we going to play out the Terri Schiavo drama? I pictured the clip on TV, playing over and over again, heard the angry voices of her parents, her ex-husband, the pious speeches of Congressmen. Not for us, I thought. But did I have a choice?

I had no time to call the children and ask their opinions. "Will you be able to take the tube out?" I asked, fearing they'd keep him alive when they ought to let him go, when he'd want to go.

"It's just for a couple of days," the doctor said in a reassuring voice.

I made the decision. "Okay." I hoped I'd made the right choice. Another load of guilt would be more than I could bear.

The nurse led the way to the family waiting room, and we all sat down. Now I thought I should call my children. I reached Michael first. He wasn't driving yet, but he said Monica would bring him to the hospital. Lori was about to leave her office. "I can't handle this," she confessed.

"It's okay. Michael is coming."

Two of the nurses left, and the charge nurse sat with me until Michael arrived. As she got up, she said, "You'll have to come up and clear out his room before you go home."

"Uh huh."

Dr. DeMarco came into the waiting room. "Mr. Z. had a blow to the head and we're checking to see if there are any after-effects. He's asleep now. Why don't you take a look at him and then go home? I'll be in the hospital tomorrow morning. Have them page me when you get here."

Michael waited while I found my way back to the Ralph's room. He was hooked up to all sorts of monitors. His forehead was stitched, and the ventilating tube was in place. I'd seen Michael fight that same tube only a couple of weeks ago; now I had to face it again. How would Ralph deal with it?

I patted his hand and left. Michael and I went upstairs to pack Ralph's things. Eyes followed us as we passed the nursing station. I was sure I heard whispers, too.

Clothing, papers, wallet, toothbrush. We tossed items haphazardly into the hospital's white paper bags.

I knew Ralph's room was needed for other patients. He couldn't have two rooms, one here and one in Intensive Care, but I felt as if we were being tossed out into the cold, as if in some vague way, we were at fault in this situation. Even as we hurried to load everything up, I felt we weren't getting done fast enough to suit the staff.

Because Michael couldn't lift the heavy bags, a nice young woman from Transportation hauled everything downstairs and helped me load the car. I'd seen her before. She'd taken Ralph down for therapy appointments at various times.

"Fallin' out of a wheelchair," she muttered to me. "Just awful. I've never heard of such a thing happening."

Michael and I stopped for dinner (Never skip meals!) at La Madeleine and then went to my house. He called Monica to bring his meds so he could spend the night. I was glad for his company, but I was too shaken to talk. We both went to bed early.

I lay in bed thinking that if this were one of my romance novels, today would be the "black moment," when all seems lost. The hero and heroine have parted, their love is threatened, life looms ahead like a black hole.

And then ...

Something happens: an event, a change of heart, a realization that life without each other is meaningless. There's a climactic scene, and they live happily ever after. And when you meet them thirty-four years later in the sequel which features their children, they are still as passionately in love as ever. Life is good. You can imagine violin music playing in the background.

Ralph and I had had our happily-ever-after. I had no confidence that this chapter would end well. The music we heard now was the beep of an IV monitor, the sound of a doctor's page, and the wail of sirens outside. With an effort, I stifled my tears and welcomed the oblivion of sleep.

The next morning I dropped Michael at his home, hurried to the hospital and after several wrong turns, found my way to Ralph's cubicle. Gowned and gloved, I patted his arm. I yearned to feel the texture of his skin, wanted him to feel the warmth of my hand, but that was impossible. We couldn't communicate verbally with the awful tube in his throat, but I could read the misery in his eyes. He tried to write me a note but succeeded only in scribbling on the page. I told him the tube would be out soon, that I'd be with him, that he would be all right. I wondered if I was lying. How could he possibly survive this horrible accident?

Hadn't he been through enough? How much more could he take?

I called Marla, who is an occupational therapist with hospital experience. She said an incident report would be filed immediately after any accident. Determined to find out exactly what had happened, I asked the doctor, a new one of course, when I could read the report. He said the head nurse would have it. I asked the nurse. She said files weren't available on weekends. On Monday I asked again. She said the patient advocate would have the information.

I called the advocacy office and asked for the bone marrow transplant advocate. *She* told me since Ralph was in Intensive Care, she couldn't help me. Upset and shaken after a three-day nightmare, I was not about to be put off. "The accident happened while he was still on the transplant floor," I reminded her.

"I'll come down and talk to you," she said. She arrived with her supervisor in tow.

He introduced himself. "How are you?" he inquired.

Did he expect me to say I was fine? Polite conversation was beyond me. "I want to know what happened to my husband," I demanded. "I want to see the accident report."

"I don't know if you can."

"How long have you worked at this hospital?"

"Quite a few years," he replied.

"And you *still* don't know?"

"Well," he said, "the person who was with your husband isn't here today. I'll talk with her and get back to you tomorrow."

"I'll call you when I get here," I said, "and I'll expect some information."

When he left, I sat by Ralph's bed and tried to breathe deeply and calm down. Not easy, when Ralph was clearly suffering.

He looked like a concentration camp inmate. Over the past months he had lost seventy-five pounds and most of his muscle mass. His legs and arms were stick-like. His hair, surprisingly, was beginning to grow in, thin wisps of gray that made him look sicker than when he was bald. The black stitches on his temple and the bruises around them were a sharp contrast to his ashen skin. Needles and tubes were attached to his body, monitors beeped as numbers flashed on and off. Surely this was hell.

The day passed in a blur. The next morning I called the Patient Advocacy office and was told the supervisor was unavailable. "He'd better be available soon," I snarled.

Five minutes later the phone rang. The supervisor cleared his throat and said, "This is a matter for Risk Management."

"Who is that?" I asked. "Your lawyers?"

"The department that deals with insurance," he answered, then added in a placating tone, "I'm going to talk to the occupational therapist who was with your husband when the accident occurred. Why don't we set up a meeting for Wednesday?"

I agreed, called Lori, and asked her to come to the meeting with me.

Then I went back to work. Someone had to be the breadwinner in our family. Besides everything else, Ralph's Medicare days had run out, and he'd nearly used up his lifetime reserve days.

The next day we had a meeting with the patient advocates from both Bone Marrow Transplant and Intensive Care, the occupational therapist, and her supervisor. I taped it.

The therapist explained that she had checked Ralph's balance before they left the floor, and it was fine; therefore she'd not belted him in. Her theory was that he had become dizzy and passed out and that caused him to fall forward.

Some weeks later I taped Ralph's memory of what happened. He said the hospital sock he wore caught in the wheel of his chair, made him lose his balance and pitch forward. Instead of grabbing *him*, the therapist grabbed the chair and this added to his forward trajectory. I wasn't surprised to hear an entirely different version of the accident.

On Wednesday afternoon Ralph's breathing tube was removed. Thank God I was spared a decision I'd dreaded having to make.

But when I arrived at the hospital, I learned there was a new development. Because of the tube, or perhaps because of something else – I never asked precisely – Ralph had developed dysphagia, inability to swallow food.

Another bodily function destroyed. This man, who had always consumed food with gusto, the spicier the better, now could not even swallow a sip of water. What other cruelties did Fate have in store for him?

In his books Rabbi Harold Kushner says he doesn't believe God deliberately punishes humankind. Accidents, illnesses, tragedies are random. In other words, life happens. But why did so many bad things have to happen to Ralph? I wondered how much courage Ralph and I had left.

I knew his swallow would be evaluated by one of the speech pathologists at the Cancer Institute. Fortunately, I knew most of the people on that staff and was sure they'd give me detailed information about a problem I knew only by name. Because I specialize in preschool and school aged children with articulation and language/learning disorders, I'd never had a patient with dysphagia and had no idea how it was treated. I was soon to learn.

Meanwhile, Ralph's condition worsened. From an offhand remark by one of the residents, I learned he had a hematoma in his brain. She said it casually, with no more thought than if she'd remarked that he had blue eyes or wore a size ten shoe.

I watched the doctors watch Ralph as they made rounds. They shut the glass sliding door to his room and huddled around his chart, glancing at him occasionally as if he were a moderately interesting fish in a large glass bowl.

He began running a fever. Saturday night he murmured sadly, "I want to go back."

"Back upstairs?"

"Back to February. Before the transplant."

I wanted to go back, too, but even farther. Back before the leukemia. Back to an ordinary, boring day. Get up, eat breakfast, read the newspaper, go to work. Nothing momentous. I'd be happy with an ordinary argument: Who gets the front page of the *Chronicle* first? What movie do we see, thriller or romance?

I'd even settle for a political argument: Ms. Moderate-to-Liberal versus Mr. Conservative.

On Sunday Ralph's fever crept upward and his oxygen level dropped alarmingly. When the night nurse came on, I asked if he could have Tylenol to lower the fever.

"I don't know."

"Isn't it in his chart?"

"I don't have time to read all that," she said. "It's two hundred pages."

Wasn't that her job, to read his chart, at least the current part? Holding my temper, I suggested, "Why don't you call the doctor?" She assented and Ralph got his dose of Tylenol.

I phoned Michael and Monica. They came and sat with me until 11:00 when Ralph's fever slowly began to drop.

His complications weren't over yet. One afternoon as I drove to the hospital, I received a call on my cell from the Intensive Care Unit fellow. "I'd like to set a time to talk to you. Mr. Zirkelbach is having some problems with his kidneys."

"I'm on the way now. What's wrong?"

"Let's not talk while you're driving. It's not an emergency."

Not an emergency? Then why not talk now? But I didn't argue. I'd be there in ten minutes. If I didn't wreck the car and kill myself on the way.

I made it. Upstairs in the ICU, I took a quick glance at Ralph (Sometimes glass windows are a good thing.) and followed the ICU fellow, an attractive young woman with long, brown hair, into a conference room.

I lowered myself into a chair and prepared to face the worst.

As I expected, the news was dire. "Your husband's kidneys are failing."

She didn't have to explain the implications. When I was burned, my own kidneys failed. Soon my arms and hands were swollen with fluid. The doctor told my parents I was terminal. Then something strange happened. I asked my mother for an apple. My father went to the store and bought one. Mother peeled the fruit and cut it into small pieces. I ate it, fell asleep, and dreamed I was climbing a hill. When I reached the top, I woke and told my mother I was better. Within the hour my kidneys began functioning again.

Months later my mother told me the story of a *refuah*, a magical food that cures illness. Although normally a realist, Mother believed this tale because one of her brothers had been gravely ill as a child in the Ukraine. Expected to die, her brother told their father that a peasant at the village market had grapes for sale and implored him to buy a bunch and bring it back to him. Although it was winter and grapes were nowhere to be had, their father went to the market and sure enough, she saw the peasant. His son did not eat the fruit but put it under his pillow. From that moment, he began to improve. By the time the grapes dried up, he was well.

Ralph would have no magical food because he could not swallow. Maybe some other miracle would happen. A miracle of modern medicine, perhaps. After all, we were in one of the world's best hospitals.

"What caused his kidney failure?" I asked the doctor.

"Well," she explained in a gentle voice, "sometimes when there's a trauma, the kidneys get angry ..."

"The kidneys '*get angry*?'" I mocked. "Talk to me like a grown-up."

She blinked at my disgust, and apologized. In adult language now, she told me Ralph's kidneys were not functioning and she recommended putting in a line for dialysis.

Another loss and more invasive treatment. "Does dialysis hurt?" I asked.

She assured me it didn't and once his kidneys began working, the treatment would stop. I heard her unspoken "if," but I agreed, as long as an experienced surgeon inserted the line. When she asked why I thought that was necessary, I described the horrible result of the lumbar puncture.

She stared at me. "I've never heard of that happening."

She had now. And she understood my fears and also my list of complaints about the Intensive Care Unit. In fact, she became one of my staunchest allies on the unit.

She suggested I speak to the current attending physician, and I did, losing my temper in the process.

"I hear how angry you are," the doctor said.

"You can't begin to imagine how angry I am," I retorted, ran over my list of grievances, and ended with, "You and the other doctors slammed the door of Ralph's room so I couldn't hear when you made rounds."

"We didn't want to disturb you."

"You didn't want us to *hear* you. Don't you ever treat my husband or me like that again."

She had no answer for that, and I went to sit with Ralph until the surgeon, a genial red-headed man, appeared.

While the surgeon inserted the dialysis line, I sat in the waiting room, picked up a novel which turned out to be a highly erotic romance, and read. When I left that night, I took the book home to finish it. I figured the hospital owed it to me.

Once dialysis began and his infections were under control, Ralph again felt better, even though his condition was still grave.

One evening he told me excitedly that some friends from the Redeemer's Baptist Church, the African-American congregation he had visited with his sister, had come to visit. "They made me a member of their church," he said.

"That was nice of them."

♦♦♦

Although Ralph was improving, my own spirits were low. One morning while I waited for his respiratory treatment to finish, I sat in the family room thumbing through a book. A few other people were scattered about the room, all of them silent, staring into space. I felt as if a heavy fog hung over us all. The room seemed as dim as my hopes for the future. I was certain Ralph was going to die.

On the way back to my office shortly afterward, I stopped at a red light, and without thinking, took my foot off the brake and rear-ended the car in front of me. My fear of a wreck had come true.

CHAPTER 23

I followed the other car into a parking lot. The driver got out but I was too shaky to stand, so I stayed behind the wheel. "I'm sorry," I said. "I wasn't paying attention. My husband is dying."

Her eyes filled with concern. Quickly, she inspected her car. "Not a scratch on it," she said, bid me goodbye and drove away.

I burst into tears and cried the rest of the way to my office. Once I pulled into the parking lot, I dried my eyes and went to work.

As the days went on, a new attending came on in the ICU. She was up-front with me and kind, and I liked her. Dr. DeMarco, my favorite bone marrow department doctor, wasn't on duty but he looked in one day, saying he'd come to check on how I was doing. I told him I was better because Ralph was better.

The physicians scheduled a care conference, with Dr. Helm present as well. Their goal, they said, was to move Ralph back to the eleventh floor as soon as possible. On the following Sunday morning I arrived at the hospital and found his cubicle empty. For an instant, my heart stopped. I stood uncertainly, glancing around the unit, afraid to enter the cubicle, afraid to ask where he was.

One of the nurses noticed my shock and came over. "He moved upstairs. Didn't someone call you?"

"No."

"Go on up."

There he was, smiling at me from the bed in a large, sunny room with a pull-down bed for me to curl up on, a closed door so no one could peer at him from outside, and nurses I knew and liked. How could a hospital room look so wonderful and welcoming? Maybe we were getting our happily-ever-after chance after all.

While Ralph was in ICU, I began eating my sack lunch in

an area called The Patio. A wide, airy space, it was filled with tables spaced far enough apart to give diners privacy. Chairs were upholstered and comfortable and made of what I supposed was fake rattan. The place had the feel of an elegant, open air restaurant one might find at a hotel or country club, except that the people seated at the tables wore surgical scrubs or other hospital garb, and many of the diners had walkers or IV poles beside them. I couldn't forget where I was, but I could relax a bit.

I continued eating there when Ralph moved upstairs. I liked the atmosphere and I wanted to avoid other patients' families on Ralph's floor. Family members and caregivers regularly share information about their loved ones' conditions, and I didn't want to discuss Ralph's situation. I feared it would depress or frighten other visitors, and truthfully, I didn't want to hear about the progress their patients were making. What I hated most was watching transplant patients ambling through the hall, doing their required exercise. I recalled Ralph striding confidently along and me panting to keep up. How different he was now, with his useless legs. I glanced away when people passed and kept to myself.

I asked the current attending physician how Ralph's wound was healing. Although the wound care specialists continued to visit him when he was in Intensive Care, the status of his pressure sore hadn't been a high priority in my mind. Now I wanted to know.

"It's better," she said, "but it's still pretty big – six inches wide and an inch deep."

All this from a needle prick. What had I done to him, signing those papers? What else *could* I have done?

I discussed this with Ralph on several occasions. Each time he seemed surprised that I gave permission for the spinal tap.

"Somebody had to do it. You couldn't."

"But why?" he asked.

"It was an emergency."

"No, it wasn't."

"It was. You weren't coherent. They thought you had encephalitis or some other serious condition."

He didn't comment, but whenever he was annoyed with me

for any reason, he glared at me and growled, "Who signed the papers?"

How would I feel, I asked myself, if our roles were reversed, if I were the one lying in bed with paralyzed legs and Ralph the one who'd scribbled his signature on the consent form for the lumbar puncture?

Wouldn't he have signed? Wouldn't he have trusted the doctor and followed medical advice?

If he had, could I forgive him? I feared the answer was no.

Had this happened a year ago or even a few months ago, I might have cratered, but I was beginning to find a core of steel deep inside. I'd weathered so much in the past year, I was now sure nothing could hurt me.

The doctor recommended that Ralph have a rectal tube, to prevent the wound being soiled by feces. Why hadn't someone suggested that months ago, before the lesion grew so large? I didn't ask, just nodded my agreement. Cliches ran through my head: You can't turn back the clock. Better late than never. But what about, a stitch in time saves nine?

One evening Ralph said casually, "You know I've gone back to being Christian."

Had he absorbed Catherine's faith along with her blood? Shocked, I said, "N...no."

"I told you."

"When?" Perhaps he had, but I didn't remember.

"When the Redeemer's Church people came."

"You said they made you a member of their church. I thought ... I thought it was honorary."

He shook his head.

A dart seemed to pierce my heart. Ralph had truly abandoned me. *I've lost the battle to Jesus,* flashed in my mind.

Ralph was ill; of course he craved the comfort of his childhood faith; he'd never become Jewish, only professed an interest in doing so in the future. But he hadn't exactly been Christian either, not during the years of our marriage.

Judaism is a religion focused on this world, not the world to come. Christianity promised him salvation in a way my faith couldn't. I could hardly begrudge him that.

Still, I felt hurt, lost. It would be many months, long after Ralph's death, before my heart caught up with my head.

Once he was back upstairs, Ralph resumed his physical and occupational therapy sessions at a more intense pace. Although he was too weak to stand or transfer to a chair by himself, he could at last move his feet. "I think I'll be home by Christmas," he said one afternoon.

Christmas seemed a long way off, but we'd already spent over five months in the hospital. What was another four, more or less?

Meanwhile, I mentioned to the doctor that I was pleased with Ralph's recovery from his mishap, but wondered why his blood counts, especially his platelets, remained so low. He agreed with my concern and said he would order a new bone marrow aspiration.

That afternoon Ralph suddenly asked, "Where do you think I should be buried?"

He couldn't be buried alongside me, in a Jewish cemetery. Knowing this, I'd always planned to be buried in our family plot in Austin.

"Iowa," I said automatically. Then his meaning hit me like a club to the head. "Why are you asking that?" I demanded.

"Because."

The doctor scheduled a conference on Saturday morning to discuss the results of the bone marrow aspiration. I didn't let myself think about it. I'd become an expert on pushing bad thoughts aside. But I did ask Lori and Michael to come with me that morning. We assembled in Ralph's room, and, with trepidation, I waited for the bone marrow results.

I wasn't prepared, never expected the doctor's words: "Mr. Zirkelbach, blasts showed up in your blood stream. You've had a relapse."

CHAPTER 24

Ralph asked quietly, "What happens now?"

"The percentage of blasts isn't high enough for a leukemia diagnosis, but since you've already had AML, we expect them to increase."

Death stared us in the face.

Ralph glanced at me. "I'd like to talk to the doctor alone."

Like sleepwalkers, we left the room and went to the family lounge. Neither of my children said a word. I sat down at the table and began to cry.

This was far worse than the original diagnosis, even though it was delivered in a much more empathetic tone. Then we'd had hope, based I'm sure on naivete, but we'd had something to cling to. Now we'd heard an undeniable truth, a death sentence.

A woman walked into the room, opened the refrigerator and turned to stare at me. She stood still, holding a cup and watching me. Hadn't she ever seen anyone cry before? Especially here, in a cancer hospital?

Finally I couldn't stand her scrutiny any longer. I jumped up and snarled, "Get out of here." When she scuttled out, I slammed the door in her face.

"Mom!" Michael said. "This is a public place."

"I don't give a damn," I answered and dropped my head into my hands.

Michael hurried out and got one of the nurses, who led us to a private conference room. After a while, she returned and said Ralph wanted us to come back.

When we walked into his room, my eyes flew to his. As if he'd lowered a mask over his face, his expression was blank.

Lori and Michael stood opposite Ralph's bed. My legs shook; I sat in the arm chair. I turned to the doctor. "I want to know if Ralph will still get dialysis and other treatments."

He looked puzzled. "Why?" I translated this to, "What's the point?"

"As far as I'm concerned, treatment can stop," Ralph said.

Horrified, I begged, "Let's talk about it."

Ralph shrugged. "Okay."

"Do you have any more questions?" the doctor inquired.

Ralph shook his head.

I had dozens – How much time, what can we do, why did this happen? – but I couldn't utter a word.

The doctor left, and the children soon followed. His face still expressionless, Ralph stared at the wall. I sat by the bed, feeling as if I'd turned to stone. I couldn't move, even to lean over and touch Ralph's hand. If I did, I might shatter into pieces. Finally I whispered, "Please don't do this."

"I'll think it over," he answered, and said no more.

We spent the weekend in silence and sorrow.

Ahead of us lay the impenetrable wall between life and death. Behind us lay all our dreams.

There were no more ifs, no maybes, only certainty.

Was I selfish, clinging to Ralph, begging him to hold on to life when the future was hopeless? Was I re-enacting Terri Schiavo's parents' scenario? "I don't want you to leave me," I sobbed one day and laid my head on his bed.

He patted my arm. "You'll be all right. You'll do something good."

His words brought me no comfort then, but they've stayed with me, and now, long after that day, I realize I want to fulfill Ralph's prediction. In the poem "When Death Comes" Mary Oliver says, "I don't want to end up simply having visited this world." I have the same wish. I hope I'll find my "something good."

Now that death was upon us, now that I was about to become the widow I'd dreaded, I forced myself to make plans. Soon I would be on my own, something I'd never had to face before. I'd been divorced once, but I'd had my parents to lean on; now I'd have to be more self-reliant. In the words of my favorite song, Ralph had always been "the wind beneath my wings." How would I fly without him?

One friend said in a knowing voice, "Your life will be different now."

That comment goes on my list of what not to say to a person

facing the death of a loved one, along with the remark by an acquaintance of my mother's a few days after my father's death: "You never get over it."

I answered my friend, "I guess things will change, but I didn't get a choice,"

I wondered how my mother felt when she became a widow. My father died at seventy-six; she lived on for another twenty-four years. The last seventeen years in the nursing home, her mind was empty of thought. What about the days before, when she lived alone in Austin? Were they empty, too? Not completely. Although she never stopped grieving for Daddy, she now took an active role in her financial affairs, meeting frequently with her trust officer and making decisions about investments.

She never expressed an interest in dating. When a man she knew asked if he could come over for the evening, she was horrified and turned him down flat.

Except for her regular visits to the bank to discuss the management of her trust, I think her days were barren without my father to care for.

I promised myself my days would be full. No matter how lonely I felt, my life would go on. I wouldn't allow widowhood to define me. There is a Yiddish proverb that says, "*Az me muz, ken men;* When one must, one can." I resolved to make that my creed.

I began to plan Ralph's funeral in his hometown and got his agreement for a memorial service at our synagogue. This was different from my mother's funeral; now I knew precisely what had to be done. Experience had taught me, but no one wants this kind of experience.

The funeral director in Iowa sent me an e-mail attachment with pictures of caskets, from unfinished pine boxes to elaborate, satin-upholstered, hermetically sealable models of polished wood trimmed in gold metal, with little pillows inside. There were even pictures on the inside of the lids – angels or flowers surrounded by curlicues of vines and leaves.

Jews are buried in coffins made of wood, which will decay quickly and allow the body to return to the earth from which it came. Mesmerized by the amenities provided for Christian dead, I scrolled through pages of more and more elaborate caskets, wondering whether grieving relatives had to take out loans to purchase them. Were these the descendants of the grave goods buried with the dead by primitive peoples or a modern way of keeping up with the Joneses?

Besides funeral plans, I had more mundane matters in mind. I asked Ralph to call his friend Darlene to do our taxes. He'd gotten an extension, and time was almost up.

Darlene expressed an interest in buying his business, and she and Ralph discussed terms. We made plans to meet in his room, and she arrived with an offer far less than what she and Ralph had decided on. Since she had all his records, I had no idea if the new offer was reasonable, and I told her I'd think it over. Her face turned red with anger. After she saw I would not back down, she gave me some unrelated (and unappreciated) advice: "Get your own post office box. You can't be taking things out of the business box."

"I use that box, too," I said.

Her response was a glare. "I need the combination to your home safe," she said next.

"*For what?*"

"I need the title to his car so it can be sold."

"No," I snapped, "you don't. I'll sell the car, and I don't give out my safe combination to anyone."

She left, furious. But I was angry, too. She may have been Ralph's pal, but she wasn't mine.

♦♦♦

Lori gave me the name of a woman, Jeanne Stevens, who might help me negotiate with the hospital about our financial situation. I hauled Ralph's medical records to her office. After reading them, she suggested she and I set up a meeting with the financial manager of the bone marrow transplant department and include Ralph's physician. Agreeing that this was a good idea, I called the appropriate financial advisor.

"That's against the law," she replied. "We can't give information to outsiders."

I called Jeanne. She immediately put her phone on conference and called the woman's supervisor, who admitted we were perfectly free to set up a meeting, but that we would need Ralph's permission to involve Jeanne. "Have him come up here and sign the papers," the departmental person said.

"He can't. He's paralyzed. Just fax the form and he'll sign it."

"We can't *fax*."

"I'm not going to fax you his signature. I just need the form and I'll bring it to you."

"She can fax it," the supervisor said.

Ralph signed the form and within a few days the patient advocate called. "This meeting you want can't be done," she said.

She'd called on my cell and I picked up while I was getting my hair cut. Aware that I was in a public place, I kept my voice low. "It's what I want."

"It can't be done. Doctors and business people don't meet."

"But that's what I want."

"I can meet with you."

Hands shaking, I said, "I'll call you back."

I never did. A little over a year after Ralph's death, I wrote the hospital president, explaining our circumstances, and the hospital wrote off the expenses incurred after his Medicare coverage ended.

By no means was everyone we dealt with so callous. The nurses on Ralph's floor were kind and helpful. They did everything possible to make him comfortable and to meet his needs. The next two attending physicians were the best of the best. Dr. DeMarco, made us cheerful just being around him; Dr. Kari, quieter and more serious, brought kindness and empathy to his patients.

We discussed Ralph's options with Dr. DeMarco. Another transplant, he said, was out of the question. Ralph was too weak, his lungs scarred by bouts of pneumonia, his kidneys just beginning to function. "He wouldn't survive." Some patients chose to get a "stem cell booster," but Dr. DeMarco said the side effects were often severe. I knew this to be true. Months ago I had met a family whose son had a booster. He developed jaundice and such tightening of the skin that he could barely move his limbs.

Additional chemo would give Ralph a month or two but would make him sick. Hi answer to that option was a definitive, "No."

I asked the doctor to let us know when the blasts multiplied enough to stop treatment, and he promised he would. He said in Ralph's case, the leukemia was advancing slowly, so we had some time. Ralph agreed to take it. Dr. DeMarco asked if Ralph preferred to go home. I promised Ralph I would make it happen if that was his wish, even though I knew he would require care far beyond what I could give. But he would be home, in his own bed, with the glass door opening onto the patio where his Monster plant grew ever larger, with his cat rubbing against him, with visits from Gabriella. Dying at home would bring peace to his last days. There'd be space for me on the king size bed beside him, and we could reach over and touch each other during the night.

The arrangements to make this work for a man who could not walk, who required a catheter, a rectal tube, a feeding tube, and constant IV medications and blood transfusions were daunting. Scary, too. Even if lifesaving treatment was discontinued, he would need round-the-clock care.

And how would I face his dying at home?

Years ago, I'd read *By Myself*, a memoir by Lauren Bacall about her life with Humphrey Bogart. One scene stuck in my mind. She recounted Bogey's dying and her horror at seeing him carried out of the house, zipped in a body bag. That scene replayed over and over in my mind until Ralph made a decision: He would not go home. He wanted to be where care was available at the push of a button. Even though he knew death was near, in the hospital he felt safe.

Nevertheless, we investigated hospice. A representative came by to talk to us. He explained that although treatments such as dialysis and the feeding tube would be discontinued, medication to control pain was available until the end. Families were encouraged to visit and spend nights at the hospice if they wished.

However, the length of stay was usually no more than two weeks. I imagined knowing in advance how much time was left, and although Ralph might not have much more than that anyway, I found the time limit hard to accept.

Michael and I made a visit to the lovely building that belonged to the hospice. It was an old mansion set back from the street and shaded by tall oak trees. I must have driven past it dozens of times and never noticed it. I clutched Michael's hand as we approached the entrance. As lovely and peaceful as it appeared, it was a house of death. Stepping inside reminded me of our first visit to the Cancer Institute's beautiful lobby. Now I believed the beauty was only skin deep.

We went inside and found the lobby deserted. Comfortable arm chairs and couches filled the room. A pot of ivy sat on the desk by the door. The sweet smell of potpourri drifted to my nose.

We ventured down the hall, saw the large dining area, with a refrigerator at one side and small tables scattered through the room. "What do you think?" I whispered.

"Nice, I guess." But I knew Michael's thoughts mirrored mine. At the stairway we paused. Michael glanced at me and I shook my head. I didn't want to intrude, nor did I want to venture any farther into the world of the dying. Even though so many mishaps had befallen Ralph in the hospital, I longed for its familiarity. The idea of Ralph traveling to this place in an ambulance was too frightening, too much like seeing him walk the last steps to an execution chamber.

As we left, Michael let out a long breath. "Well?" he said once we were back in the car.

"No. It would be a nice place to live. But," my voice broke, "it's a place to die."

I described the hospice to Ralph, trying to emphasize how peaceful it was, but I was relieved when he said he did not want to move there.

The hospital also had a hospice program, but its duration was only two days. Moving Ralph one floor up, with new nurses, new room, even new doctors for the last two days of his life, whenever that would be, seemed cruel.

The nurse from the transplant floor told us they could provide "comfort care." That was the best – or the least heart-wrenching – choice.

And so Ralph's hospital room became our home. Here we shared our thoughts and remembered better times. I wish I had asked Ralph what he believed about death. We'd spoken about it many times, always in the abstract, and he'd said he believed in an afterlife. Did he still? I didn't ask, but I thought his Christianity gave him that assurance.

He accepted his fate. I think he welcomed it. An active person, how could he live encumbered by a wheelchair? How could he enjoy meals, deprived of the spicy food he loved? When I asked him if he'd like me to bring back his computer, he shook his head. "That's in the past."

One day I said wistfully, "I wish we could take another trip," and he answered, "It's okay. I take trips in my head."

Surprisingly, his interest in current events revived, and although he said that watching TV was difficult, he questioned the nurses and chatted with the doctors about what was going on in the world.

I wish I could have been as accepting as Ralph of what awaited him. One day I asked, "Now that you've gone back to Christianity, does this mean we won't be together in a future life?"

Why did I ask this? For me, death seemed a black hole. I never pictured Elysian Fields, streets of gold, heavenly choirs. I remember being touched by Robert Browning's "Prospice:" "Oh, thou soul of my soul, I shall clasp thee again..." But I never quite believed it.

Ralph shrugged at my question. "I guess not."

Stunned, hurt beyond all measure, I turned away so he wouldn't see my tears. In his mind, he wasn't just leaving me for a while; he was leaving for eternity ... if there was an eternity.

Death was my greatest fear. I felt the same emotions as Robert Burns when the poet addresses death as

Thou unknown Almighty
Cause of all my hope and fear...

I remember when I first became aware that someday I would die. I was seven, and one hot summer afternoon my neighborhood friend Lynn and I ran out of things to do. "Let's play dead," she suggested.

"Okay. How?"

"Just lie down on the walk and cross your hands over your heart and shut your eyes."

I followed her lead, felt the hard, hot pavement beneath me, the sun behind my closed lids, and the stillness of the July afternoon. I was terrified. "Dead" meant being as still as the stony walkway. I sat up, gazed at Lynn, lying with her bare feet almost touching mine and a satisfied smile on her face. Why was she smiling? Death was scary, not pleasant. But perhaps Lynn, a Christian, had been introduced to death in a different, more hopeful way. For Jewish children, death is a taboo subject.

That evening I was filled with anxiety and I began to cry. Unwilling to confess the reason, I said I had a stomach ache. And I did – the fluttering pain that comes from fear.

For months afterward, I was afraid to cross my hands over my heart. Even as an adult, I was terrified by the great mystery of death, by the thought that dying must be done alone. Ralph did not share my fears. His religion comforted him, but it left a gulf between us.

CHAPTER 25

As August wound to a close, we awaited a visit from Ralph's family. His mother, severely bent by arthritis, planned to accompany his sisters, and Ralph looked forward to seeing them one more time. He promised to wait until after their visit and one from my cousins the following week before making a decision to stop the treatments that kept him alive.

I cherished every day we had left. Even when we didn't talk, I felt a comfort in his presence, a bittersweet tenderness. In the darkest of our bleak times, stars twinkled through.

A few days before the visitors arrived, I told Ralph, "I don't want your family to talk to me about religion." I feared, under the circumstances, their efforts to convert me might become overt.

"If they do, just walk out," Ralph suggested.

"That would be rude."

"Then tell them you don't want to talk about it."

"They're your family. You tell them."

Finally he agreed. Maybe he told them, maybe not, but the subject of religion did not come up.

They arrived on Lori's birthday, August 28.

The months of August and September are the peak of hurricane season, and a storm was brewing in the Caribbean. Her name was Katrina. We worried about thunderstorms interfering with travel, but the family arrived without mishap.

As the hurricane passed over Florida into open water, it gathered strength. The storm headed toward Louisiana. Now that everyone was safely here, we didn't take much notice. Hurricanes are a part of late summer on the Gulf Coast and unless one of them is predicted to make landfall in our area, Houstonians pay little mind.

We spent time visiting. Ralph's mother and sisters sprawled in chairs in Ralph's hospital room as if it were the family living room and reminisced about incidents from Ralph's childhood.

"Kate, remember the time I hooked up the phone to a

loudspeaker?" Ralph asked.

"So you could broadcast my conversations – my *private* conversations – with my boyfriend all through the house. How could I forget?" his sister answered.

"And remember when I stayed with you in Kingsville for a summer?" Sara added. "You were stricter than Dad."

"You needed someone strict," Ralph said.

As a youngster Sara was the family rebel. Apparently she didn't outgrow it. During a chat about Iowa politics, she leaned over to me and whispered, "Thelma, I have something to tell you. I'm a Democrat." In her family this was rebelliousness in the extreme.

Catherine and I talked about the fun we'd had when she came to donate her stem cells, and she said if Ralph chose to have another transplant, she'd donate again.

If only he could make that choice.

By the time they'd been here a day, Ralph's mother had made friends with other families and with the hospital staff, Catherine had donated to the blood bank, and they'd made Ralph smile. We had a family dinner at Pappasito's, a nearby Tex-Mex restaurant, while Gabriella charmed her relatives. Our only sorrow was that Ralph couldn't enjoy the food and laughter with us.

While we enjoyed ourselves, the news from the outside world was grim. Hurricane Katrina churned toward New Orleans and as Monday, August 29, wore on, we heard that the city had been devastated when the levees gave way. Scenes of terrified victims, flooded streets, buildings and houses filled the TV screen. New Orleans looked like a war zone. Along with everyone else in the country, we were shocked.

Houston came to the rescue of New Orleans' newly homeless, turning the old Astrodome into a huge shelter. Ralph, who heard this through the hospital grapevine, told me they were bringing criminals to Houston. I didn't believe that, but instead of driving past the Dome on my way home at night as usual, I began taking another route. People jammed into a crowded space might not be criminals, but violence could erupt in those surroundings and I took no chances.

I heard from Dr. DeMarco that several transplant patients

were airlifted to the Cancer Institute and were now on the eleventh floor. Our synagogue school enrolled temporary students whose families had fled their homes in New Orleans.

After Ralph's family said their last goodbyes, we sat quietly, knowing we would not all be together again. My heart ached for Ralph's mother. Twice I had almost lost my son, and I knew too well the pain in her heart.

Ralph and I looked forward to the next weekend, when my cousins Bruce and Bonnie and their daughter Valerie with whom I was so close would arrive. They flew in on Sunday and came straight to the hospital. Ralph was delighted with the company. Bruce, my first cousin, who looks years younger than sixty-five, is a great joke teller, and he kept Ralph amused with political jokes and anecdotes about the chain of beauty/barber shops he owned. Bonnie, his dark-haired, soft-spoken wife, chimed in, adding stories about her cooking failures. "I'll use those in the book I'm finishing," I said. "My heroine doesn't like to cook."

Ralph worried continually that I would not make my mid-September book deadline because of his illness, or worse, his death. I assured him I'd finish the book, and if not, my editor would certainly give me an extension. I think he vowed to keep himself alive somehow until the manuscript was in my publisher's hands.

Valerie asked me if Ralph had seen a counselor. I laughed and told her that soon after his transplant a doctor had paid him a visit. Ralph answered her questions gruffly and later interrogated Lori and me as to which of us had asked for the consult. Neither of us; a psychiatric visit is standard after transplant.

Valerie asked permission to talk to Ralph's doctor. Because Dr. Kari was his attending for the first time and I didn't know him well, I suggested she call Dr. DeMarco. She did, and liked the personable physician as much as we did.

On Tuesday I looked forward to the farewell dinner we planned at Trevisio's, a lovely restaurant in the Medical Center. I worked with my morning kids and drove home for lunch, feeling, if not hopeful, at least better than usual.

And then my cell phone rang.

"Dr. Kari would like to talk with you."

"Yes, he mentioned that when we met Sunday," I said. "How about tomorrow afternoon?"

"No, now," the nurse said.

"But ..."

"Your husband has had a turn for the worse. He's having trouble breathing."

My heart spiraled down to my toes. "I'll be there in fifteen minutes."

All the way to the medical center I tried to prepare for the event no one is ever prepared for. As I drove, I told myself, *"You have to face this sometime. You will be strong."* And, *"You will drive carefully. You will not have a wreck."* If I did, I'd be too late.

I pulled up to the hospital, thrust my keys into the valet's hand, and raced through the lobby. At least eight elevators served this part of the hospital and all of them seemed to be somewhere else. Clenching my hands, I waited, and finally an elevator door slid open.

Upstairs I hurried to Ralph's wing. A nurse stopped me as I passed the nursing station. "It's all right. He's okay now."

Another rush of adrenaline but this time from relief. "What happened?"

"His nurse is in the room. She'll fill you in."

When I opened the door, Ralph waved weakly. He wore an oxygen mask, and he was chalky white.

"It was more a scare than anything," the nurse said. "We gave him steroids and he's much better now."

In the aftermath of fear, Ralph was exhausted. "Shall I call Valerie and tell them not to come today?" I asked, and he nodded.

I was worn out, too. I wanted to hold Ralph's hand to reassure myself he was still with me.

"The doctor would like to talk with you," the nurse reminded me. "He'll meet with you in the family lounge. He's about finished seeing patients."

The doctor, a dark-skinned man of medium height, came into the family room and sat across from me. He didn't have Dr.

DeMarco's smiling good nature, but his brown eyes filled with concern. "I want to get to know you a little bit and learn about your wishes," he began.

I was certain "your wishes" meant, "How do you want us to proceed when death seems inevitable?'

"Ralph has a do not resuscitate order," I said, "and I want to honor that. I want to know when the blast count goes up or the blood counts go low enough so that treatment should stop. He doesn't want to be kept alive once that happens."

The doctor nodded. "I'll talk to you when it's time."

"I guess today wasn't the time," I said. "He seemed upset, and I don't think he will be when ... when the ... the final moment comes."

"I agree. And we'll work together." He seemed the kind of person we'd like to know as a friend, and I felt Ralph was fortunate to have him as attending physician now.

I went back to Ralph's room, pulled down the Murphy bed and lay down. We spent a quiet afternoon. My cousins peeked in to say goodbye in the evening, and then I went with them to Trevisio's, where Lori joined us and we watched the sun set over the medical center.

The weekend after they left, Ralph was in a talkative mood, reminiscing about his adventures growing up. "Kate and I and some of the neighborhood kids had a secret club," he said. "We met in a shed in our back yard. One day we found a note there, saying the writer knew about our club. We couldn't figure out who it was. A few days later we found another note and then another."

"Did you ever find out who sent them?"

"Yep, finally she confessed. They were from my mother."

I couldn't picture Ralph's mother writing notes to tease her kids, but then I thought of the twinkle in her eye and decided I could. My mother might have spied on a club but she'd never have written notes.

Ralph told me about a boy in the neighborhood who bullied him. "Then I found out he was afraid of snakes. I caught one and took it over to his house and told him if he didn't leave me alone, I'd set the snake on him. He never bullied me again.

"And another time, I grabbed a note this guy in my class wrote to his girlfriend. He chased me home from school, and when I passed a mailbox, I dropped it in."

"Did he catch you and beat you up?"

"Nope. I guess he was too busy trying figure out how to get his note out of the mailbox."

We reminisced about trips we'd taken: to Chile to see Haley's Comet, to Oaxaca for a solar eclipse, to England and Greece. We talked about Ralph's favorite childhood pet, a crow named Blackie who stole the neighbors' clothespins. We talked about Ralph's cooking, about my upcoming book, about our kids. We recalled the time a pipe had broken and our breakfast room ceiling had caved in. We recalled the jokes and oxymorons we'd laughed over together through the years. That afternoon conversation is one of my dearest memories.

Now I thought I knew the meaning of love. It's laughing together, sharing a mega-box of popcorn at a movie, resting your cold feet against a warm back on a winter night. It's the scent of your lover's skin, the whisper of his breath, the hand that leads you through a dark night. These, too, I would remember.

I no longer wanted to write an expose of the medical world. Nothing could undo what happened to Ralph. I would find another way to record Ralph's final year and to celebrate his life.

Ralph wished he could see Gabriella one last time. She could not come onto the transplant floor, but Dr. DeMarco, now back on the floor, promised Ralph could meet her in the lobby the following weekend.

On that Sunday afternoon Ralph, very frail now, was transferred to a chair with a wooden head rest. He was belted in and, accompanied by Michael and a nurse, we took the elevator down to the lobby. The nurse left us near one of the entrances to wait for Monica and the children.

Across the room near another entry, a family of three huddled. The woman sobbed loudly, fiercely. Remembering the woman in the family room who intruded on my grief, I turned my back to give this family privacy. My heart ached for her. Without knowing her specific circumstances, I knew how she felt.

On the other side of the lobby a volunteer manned a popcorn cart. The smell wafted to my nose and made me long for happier times.

In a few minutes, Monica, Marco, and Gabriella arrived. Gabriella skipped across the lobby, eyes sparkling. "Popo, how do you feel?"

Ralph smiled tenderly at her. "Okay."

Marco, always reserved, came to Ralph's side and shook his hand.

Ralph and Gabriella talked for a few minutes, and then the popcorn vendor caught her attention. "Can I get some?"

Ralph's eyes followed as Marco took her over to the cart. He would not enjoy her presence again, would miss the chance to see her grow up. It was a wrenching moment for all of us.

I glanced at Michael. His eyes were full of tears.

Our visit lasted no more than fifteen minutes. By the end, Ralph was exhausted, his head leaning back against the head rest. We said goodbye, and the nurse wheeled him to the elevator. He took a last look at Gabriella. "I hope she'll remember me," he said wistfully.

"She will." I promised myself I'd make sure of that.

She hasn't forgotten. Just last week when she came to spend the evening with me, she said, "If I had one wish in the world, Nana, I would wish for Popo to come back."

Touched by her eight-year-old sincerity, I said, "Popo hoped you wouldn't forget him."

She looked surprised. "How could I forget Popo?" she asked. "I loved him."

CHAPTER 26

The following week a new storm loomed in the Gulf. Her name was Rita. After the devastation of Katrina, with much of New Orleans reduced to rubble, people along the Gulf were nervous.

With my focus on Ralph, I didn't pay attention to the forecasts, so I was surprised on Wednesday when the talk in the synagogue school teachers' lounge was all about evacuating. I called Lori when I got home. "What should we do?" I asked, too overwhelmed with Ralph's situation to make a decision on my own. "Maybe I could come to your house."

"No," she said. "The big tree by my bedroom window could fall down in a hurricane. Your house is safer."

"All right. We'll stay here."

I hung up, and a few minutes later the phone rang. "Thelma, this is Thelma." My cousin from San Antonio, both of us named for our grandmother, was calling. "They say that hurricane is on its way to Houston," she said. "Why don't you come and stay with us in San Antonio?"

"Let me call my daughter. I'll call you back."

Despite the talk at school, I didn't believe we needed to panic. I'd lived through many near-misses when hurricanes were predicted to slam into our part of the Gulf Coast and turned away.

Of course, I'd also lived through a hit. In 1983 Hurricane Alicia roared right into us. The day before, I'd told our new speech pathologist who'd moved here from Kansas that Houston was too far inland for a storm to batter; then I'd wakened in the middle of the night to the howl of wind. The lashing rain and pounding wind lasted for hours. When the eye passed over, Ralph and I slipped outside on our front porch and stood in the eerie silence, then hurried back inside to safety.

Now I vacillated. Stay or leave? I called Lori, who was emphatic. "No. I don't want to get out on the highway." We didn't accept my cousin's invitation.

That evening Lori and I talked again and discussed our

options.

"What if something happens to Ralph and I can't get to the hospital?" I said. "I want to stay there."

"All right. I'll bring my cats and stay at your house. My friend Pat can come with me. She's cat-sitting for another friend. That'll make five cats. Is it okay?"

"Sure. What's a couple of cats more or less? Just keep them separated."

Lori agreed. She'd come over the next afternoon.

I drove to the Kroger's where I usually shopped, foolishly thinking I could pick up some bottled water and canned food for Lori and her friend. The shelves were virtually empty. Not a bottle of water was left. I picked up some tuna fish and a can of unappetizing Vienna sausages. That would have to be sufficient.

When I got home, my mother-in-law called. "Does Ralph know about the storm?" she asked.

"Of course," I said. "If he doesn't have the television on, he's heard it from the staff."

"Is he worried?"

"Ralph never worries," I assured her and she hung up to give him a call.

The next morning I dragged chairs and plants off the patio and pushed the garbage can into the garage. The day was a typical September scorcher with bright, clear skies. One would never imagine that a storm lurked in the Gulf of Mexico.

I worked in fits and starts, my body soaked with sweat. Heat was dangerous. A third of my skin was grafted when I was burned, and since then I hadn't been able to get rid of heat through perspiration. When I get overheated, I pass out. *Please, not now,* I thought.

After I gathered in everything I could lift, I packed, cramming clothes, important papers and books into an overnight bag. Crackers, peanut butter and jelly went into a plastic bag. Midway through the afternoon Ralph called. "You need to get over here. They're locking down the hospital."

"I'm not ready."

"I'll tell the nurse to call downstairs and give the security guard your name. Hurry."

I showered, changed and hauled my things out to the car. As I drove away, I wondered if my house would be standing when I returned. *Don't think about it. There's nothing you can do.*

Not surprisingly, the parking garage was full when I reached the Medical Center. What if I had to park on the roof? Goodbye, car. Fortunately, after driving up and down the rows for about twenty minutes, I found a space just down the last ramp from the roof.

The elevator was a long walk from my parking space. My suitcase had wheels, but I had to lug my bag of food. At the hospital door, the security guard asked for the room number I was visiting, checked my ID, and snapped a plastic bracelet around my wrist. They were serious about the lockdown, the guard said. Anyone without a wristband would be told to leave.

Upstairs I unpacked while every few minutes the TV blared the latest coordinates of the storm. Out in the hall after getting settled, I chatted with the mother of the patient next door to Ralph. She told me only one family member per room could stay. She was leaving; her husband would remain with their daughter. I guessed if they didn't set limits, the building would be filled to overflowing with overnight "guests."

The nurse dropped off a paper explaining how the hospital would operate during the storm. The cafeteria would continue serving, but with a limited menu. A full staff of nurses, aides, and doctors would be in the building. No one was to go outside. In fact, when I went down to dinner a bit later, I saw that the doors were barricaded and the lobby deserted. And the sun still shone.

A sense of the surreal pervaded the cafeteria, as guests and staff, all adorned with ID wrist bands, filled the tables and "dined" on the unappetizing roast beef provided for the evening meal. There was little conversation. All eyes were trained on the television monitors, all ears attuned to the meteorologists whose faces filled the screens, whose ominous voices we strained to hear. "The path of probability for Hurricane Rita indicates it may hit squarely in the Houston-Galveston area." Murmurs of apprehension hummed through the room whenever these dire predictions sounded.

Later that evening when I was already dozing, Ralph's nurse came in, leaned over my bed and pulled the window blinds down. "Safety precaution," she explained.

The next morning we turned on the TV to shocking news. Highways leading out of Houston were like the proverbial "parking lots," jammed with cars that barely moved. Heat, humidity, and traffic collided dangerously. Pictures of angry, frustrated drivers and their passengers flashed across the screen. Service stations ran out of gas because trucks could not get through. We heard that High Occupancy Vehicle lanes were slated to open so cars could *move*, but as hours crept by, those lanes remained closed.

A bus filled with residents of a Houston area nursing home overturned near Dallas. Many of the elderly people aboard the bus were killed.

The storm inched closer. Calls came from friends and relatives across the country. Was the wind blowing? No. Were we all right? Yes. Were we afraid? No. And what was the point, anyway? We could do nothing but wait and listen to the endless weather reports. We both fell asleep, Ralph because he was getting weaker ... and me, well, I remembered drowsing through much of Hurricane Alicia and concluding that the low barometric pressure made me sleepy.

When I woke the next morning, I lifted the blind a few inches and peeked out. The early morning sky was gray, a few drops of rain splashed against the window pane, but the trees below were still. Nevertheless, anxiety hung in the air as the city waited for Rita to strike.

The day wore on. The skies grew cloudier but there was little rain, no wind. Still, we knew the storm was imminent.

I wished Ralph and I could have another conversation, but he wasn't up to it.

Then in the evening, a few hours before the predicted landfall, Rita turned northeast. Tension mounting, fingers crossed, we watched the weather reports until we knew the storm would miss our city.

Rita slammed into the Beaumont-Port Arthur area and never made it to Houston. You could almost feel the long sigh of relief that traveled through the hospital.

Saturday dragged by with news stories about the wind damage in Beaumont. We still worried about the aftermath of the storm here, the possibility of tornados or heavy rains, but nothing happened. On Sunday, evacuees, some of whom had spent fourteen hours on drives that normally took no more than three, wearily headed back to Houston.

Sunday afternoon I went home from the hospital. The city looked like a movie set without the actors. Neighborhoods were deserted, with little traffic on the streets, gas stations and supermarkets closed, few people to be seen. But Houston had been lucky. I could have been seeing downed trees, broken glass, damaged homes.

I turned down our street, thankful to see everything as usual. My house still stood, the pine tree beside it straight and tall, the crepe myrtle in the front garden bedecked with pink flowers. When I opened the door, the cats raced up to me, meowing their greetings, rubbing against my legs.

Lori told me there was a brief power outage, long enough for everything in my freezer to spoil. We hauled half-thawed chicken and hamburger patties to the trash.

In a proactive move, I had baked a cake to be served after Ralph's memorial service. Embarrassed at having done this, I dumped the cake in the trash without mentioning to Lori what it was for.

Since we had no frozen entrees left, Lori and I set out to find a place to eat dinner. We found the Lemongrass Cafe, a delightful and quiet Asian fusion restaurant not far from home. We said little during the meal, both of us tired from the tense weekend.

When school opened several days later, I heard stories of families flying to Los Angeles or New York, fleeing to Dallas, Austin, San Antonio. Everyone had something to tell. Everyone was greatly relieved at our miraculous escape from harm.

Later that week the Communication Disorders Alumni Association at the University of Houston, of which I was past president, held a symposium. The current board president had called me several weeks earlier to tell me they planned to present Ralph with a plaque to thank him for his contributions to the board. I was thrilled, and so was he when I told him. He had been board president as much as I, listening patiently to my concerns, formatting the program for our 2004 wine tasting, even making coffee for a graduation reception.

On Saturday I thanked the board in Ralph's name, not only for the plaque but for their support during his long illness.

The plaque read: "We offer this token of our love and appreciation to Ralph Zirkelbach in recognition of his many years of support and service to the University of Houston Communication Disorders Alumni Association." We put it on the window sill in Ralph's hospital room.

During the following week Ralph realized he had not had his new will notarized. Fortunately the hospital had a notary on staff, and we completed this task easily.

One afternoon I heard from Lori. "Someone down the hall died while I was visiting Ralph," she said, her voice shaking. "His wife was crying and screaming so loudly, you could hear her all through the wing. It really upset me."

I remembered my father suffering a cardiac arrest a few nights before he died. My mother wailed, "Oh God, take me instead, take me." I remembered her screams and swore to myself I wouldn't do that. "I won't make a scene," I told Lori. "I promise."

I made a decision that day: I would not wait to clean out Ralph's room. I didn't think I could handle putting his things into bags and taking them home ... after. I quietly began removing a few items at a time.

At home, I baked another cake.

I made one more promise to myself: Ralph would not be alone when he died. My father was in Intensive Care when he died. The hospital where he was a patient did not allow family members to visit in the ICU except at specified times. Once when we visited Daddy, he peered at us, confused, and asked, "Where have you all been?"

I vowed Ralph would not have to ask that question.

I suppose, to outward appearances, I was "ready." But not in my heart. Is anyone ready to say the final goodbye?

CHAPTER 27

I spent the following weekend at the hospital. Seven weeks had passed since we learned the leukemia had returned. Ralph had lived thirty-five more days, and he didn't seem to be suffering. I thanked God for every moment.

Although Ralph wasn't in pain, he was weak and no longer felt like talking; so I spent some of my time reading a book by Jodi Piccoult, *Her Sister's Keeper*, in which the main character, an adolescent girl, was conceived as a donor for her sister, who has leukemia. Perhaps not the best kind of book to be reading now, but the story was riveting.

When the emotions of the story overwhelmed me, I watched baseball on TV. That season the Houston Astros had a dismal start, but suddenly in August they made a surprising turnaround and propelled themselves into the National League playoffs. Now they faced their old nemesis, the Atlanta Braves.

Again, sports distracted me. Watching ballgames gave me surcease from the constant despair of Ralph's illness, the awful reminder that his days were running out. I wanted the Astros to win, to give me something to cheer about.

Sunday noon I watched the beginning of the ballgame from home. The Astros fell behind, so I went to the grocery store. Ralph often chided me for being a fair-weather fan, but I wasn't in the mood to watch a loss. At the checkout counter, I glanced at my watch. I wanted to get to the hospital as soon as possible, and I couldn't help fretting over the snail's pace of the line.

Suddenly the woman in front of me, cell phone at her ear, screamed. Every customer within earshot, and there were many of us, stared at her in horror. Then she shouted, "Lance Berkman hit a home run with the bases loaded," and everyone relaxed. Several customers added their shouts to hers.

I went home, stashed my groceries and headed for the hospital. Michael joined me in Ralph's room. While Ralph dozed, we watched the remainder of the Astros/Braves game, which was tied in the bottom of the ninth … and tenth … and fourteenth … and …

Michael left. I lay on the Murphy bed, absorbed in the game. In the bottom of the eighteenth, young Chris Burke came to bat. Not by a long shot did anyone expect him to get a hit, let alone the winning hit. But he smashed a home run into the stands. And the fans went wild.

On to the Cardinals and the National League Championship Series. When the Astros beat St. Louis, the Chronicle headline, shouted in double-sized font, "Houston, We Have a Pennant."

Although Ralph paid no attention to baseball – he'd never been a sports fan anyway – that Sunday marked one more precious day together.

This was Ralph's second week with Dr. DeMarco as his attending. Our favorite physician's being on the floor didn't change Ralph's prognosis, but his presence cheered us both. I recall word for word the original diagnosis by Dr. Riker, but it is Dr. DeMarco and others as compassionate as he, whose memories I cherish.

During Tuesday rounds Dr. Helm appeared. Dr. DeMarco had been invited to China for a consultation and would be gone the rest of the week.

On Tuesday afternoon Dr. Helm sent word down that she would like to see me. We met in the hallway outside Ralph's door. "Your husband is very ill now. It won't be long," she said gently.

My lips felt numb as I asked, "When?"

"This week, I think. I'm sorry."

The next morning when I had gathered myself, I suggested to Ralph that he call Darlene. Our income tax extension would be over on the fifteenth and I wanted to be sure our tax return was completed. He called and they chatted for a few minutes. He asked about the taxes but didn't seem to be getting a specific answer.

I signaled to him to hand me the phone. "Can I pick up our tax return on Saturday?" I asked.

"No, you cannot pick up your tax return on Saturday," she replied in the tone one might use to a feeble-minded child. "I haven't even begun yours yet. I have clients, you know."

Excuse me. I thought we were clients, too. But I didn't say that because I would not argue with her in front of Ralph. No matter that I found her obnoxious, I knew her friendship was important to him and to his business. Instead I said, "Well, our situation has changed and that may affect our time table. I'll call you back and we can discuss it." I took my cell phone out in the hall and dialed her number.

When she answered, I said, "Ralph's doctor told me he's going to die very soon. I thought you might want to take that into account."

"Do you think *I* need a *doctor* to tell me he's dying? I can see that for myself." Her voice dripped sarcasm.

"Don't you need his signature for the tax return?"

"Of course not. You should know better."

I'd never heard such venom. "Don't you talk to me like that," I snapped.

"You know," she said, "you're a very poor communicator."

Could she have thought of a nastier thing to say to a person whose profession is communication? "Call me when the return is ready," I said and hung up. Shaking, I walked back into Ralph's room. Then I burst into tears.

"What's wrong?" he asked.

"Your friend is a bitch."

"She doesn't like you. Get over it."

"Why doesn't she like me?" I sniffled.

"You're female. She doesn't like women. I mean it. Get over it."

For Ralph's sake, I did. But Darlene had only begun her nastiness. When she finally did finish the taxes, several weeks after Ralph's death, she informed me she'd closed Ralph's business. I was stunned. She'd taken it upon herself to shut down someone else's company. Only after months of negotiations through our lawyers did I learn she'd lost almost all Ralph's clients within the first month after she'd taken over his accounts and the business she'd "closed," was virtually non-existent.

Wednesday passed. Ralph got weaker, an infection ravaging his body.

On Wednesday evening Yom Kippur began. Another Kol

Nidre. Another day to atone for sins. A passage in the holiday prayer book, a quotation from Yedaya Penini says,

And remember that the companionship of time is but of short duration. It flies more quickly than the shades of evening. We are like a child that grasps in his hand a sunbeam. He opens his hand soon again, but to his amazement, finds it empty and the brightness gone.

This was on my mind as I marked the end of a year of sorrow, with more sorrow to come.

The hospital provided a service via TV for its Jewish patients, and of course there were services at the synagogue, but I couldn't bring myself to go there, to sit alone, to remember the last Yom Kippur and the sore throat that began this descent into the dark. So instead of taking my sorrows and fears to God, I hid from Him and pretended Yom Kippur didn't exist. I spent the day by Ralph's side, the place where I belonged anyway.

When Ralph's ordeal began, we had had such hopes, such certainty. Someone remarked to me a year later that families have no idea of the financial toll cancer causes. But the emotional burden is much heavier.

That Thursday I held Ralph's hand. It was warm, life still pulsing through his veins. For a little while. But I felt him slipping away from me, hovering on the threshold between life and death. I wanted to pull him back; I wanted to let him go, to wish him Godspeed, to let him find rest and peace.

CHAPTER 28

Friday morning Lori had dental surgery. I dropped her off at the oral surgeon's office on Interstate 10, a forty-five minute drive from the hospital. Several hours later I went back to get her. She was woozy but all right, so I left her at her house and headed for the hospital.

A friend had given me the name of an attorney who specialized in estates. Michael and I were to meet with him at 3:30 that afternoon. I hated to leave Ralph again, but this appointment was urgent and after spending some time with Ralph, I headed out.

The day was hot and muggy, more like August than October. Jiggling my keys, I walked to the garage and pressed the elevator button for the sixth floor. The door opened and I went to my car.

I couldn't find it.

I thought I'd parked on six but I must have made a mistake. I trudged back to the elevator and went to seven. No car. I walked up and down the aisle, tried six again, then five and on down. Several silver Toyota Camrys were parked on various floors, but none of them was mine. Hot and frustrated, I called Michael and told him my dilemma.

"Cancel the appointment," he suggested.

"I don't think I should."

"Call and say the doctor wants to talk to you and ask if you can come later. Don't say you lost your car."

"Right." If I told the truth, they'd think I was a nut case. We rescheduled for 4:00.

I kept walking through the garage, getting hotter and hotter, and more and more upset. Finally I went to the main floor and called security. By the time they arrived I was soaked with perspiration and practically in tears. And it was nearly 4:00.

As we drove slowly through the garage, I called Michael and the attorney's office and postponed the appointment again.

"Someone maybe trying to repossess your car?" the parking guard asked in a friendly tone.

"Huh? No, of course not. It's paid for. I just can't find it. My ... my husband's really sick."

"Don't you worry. If it's here, we'll find it."

We did. I have no idea what floor it was on, but there it was. I'm sure I'd passed the darned auto ten times in my search. I thanked my rescuer and got in. By now it was past 4:30.

Never having been to the attorney's office, I got lost. I had to call the receptionist to talk me to the right street.

Michael was already in the waiting room when I shuffled in. Jeff Hall, a tall gray-haired man, with a friendly smile, welcomed us and led us into the airy conference room.

Shoving my sweaty hair out of my face, I explained our situation. Ralph's business affairs were a tangled web of corporate entities. Closing the sale of his Iowa farm, which had been scheduled for that day, had been postponed until the following week. Our charges at the hospital were increasing by the minute.

"I've heard tales a lot worse," Jeff said smiling. "Let's take a look at the will."

I handed it over.

"Uh oh," he said, scanning the document. "Not good."

That was the last thing I expected to hear. "What's wrong?"

"Well, he's got different witnesses on the final page than on this page," he said, tapping his finger on the paper. "That won't fly."

My heart fell. "What do we need to do?"

"We can fix it this evening. I'll send one of our staff and the notary to the hospital if you can get another witness, maybe a friend."

I called Marla, and she said she'd be happy to meet us. "Then we'll go out to dinner. You need some nourishment," she said. That sounded like a good idea. Not that I'd missed any nourishment, but I did need a stress-free hour.

Jeff rounded up his two staff members. I was so relieved that this problem, which would have nullified Ralph's will, was easily remedied and that Jeff could get it done immediately, that I could barely believe my luck in finding this kind attorney.

The two young men followed me to the hospital, parked and met me in the lobby. "Wow," said one of them as we passed the grand piano, "no wonder your medical bills are so high."

Marla met us upstairs. Ralph stared, not quite comprehending who all these visitors were. The paralegal explained and asked him if he understood and was signing of his own accord.

"Yes," he managed.

He picked up the pen, but his hand was too weak to write.

"Here, Ralph. Let me position your hand," Marla said.

"She's an occupational therapist," I explained to the legal people. "She does this all the time."

Marla guided Ralph through his signature, then she and the paralegal signed, the notary added his signature and seal, and we were done.

"I'm taking Thelma to dinner," Marla said to Ralph.

"Will you be back?" he asked me, looking worried.

"In an hour."

"Promises, promises," he said in a teasing voice so like his normal self that I blinked.

I leaned down and gave him a hug. "I'll see you soon." Marla and I had a quiet dinner at the Stables, a nearby steak restaurant and a Houston institution. With iced tea, we toasted the fact that we'd gotten Ralph's will taken care of; we talked about movies and books, anything but the moment looming closer and closer.

Back at the hospital I saw Dr. Helm, who said, "I think twenty-four hours."

I swallowed and leaned against the wall. *Too soon.*

Ralph was glad to see me back. While I was telling him about my disappearing car and the dinner with Marla, the phone rang. It was his younger brother Louis.

Ralph was too weak to lift the receiver, so I positioned it for him and he listened to Louis for a few moments, and then said his final goodbye to his brother.

Even though Dr. Helm told me to expect the end, I couldn't process her words. I couldn't really accept that Ralph was going to leave this earth, leave me.

When I was getting ready for bed, the nurse, a sweet Filipino lady who seemed to genuinely like Ralph, suggested we leave the hall door open so the staff could look in often. A good idea. Germs from outside didn't matter any more.

"I'm going to sleep now," I said to Ralph. "Do you want anything?"

He shook his head and looked at me intently. With great effort, he said, "I... love ... you."

Those were his last words to me.

With the door open, the room was cold, and I asked for extra blankets and huddled under them. Even with a sleeping pill, I woke every little while to reassure myself that Ralph was all right.

The next day, true to my nature, I counted hours. Dr. Helm had said twenty-four. Maybe she was wrong.

Ralph slept most of the day, only waking when the nurses came to check his vital signs. I went home to get clean clothes and to put food in the cats' bowls, and then I returned to sit next to Ralph, resting my head on his arm, patting his hand, telling him I loved him but no longer hearing a response.

He was weaker, his body shutting down. He was getting ready to die.

And so I waited. I was glad no one came to visit. I wanted our last hours to be for just the two of us. Even though Ralph couldn't or didn't communicate with me, I was certain he knew I was beside him.

At 9:00 p.m. I noted that Dr. Helm's twenty-four hours had passed and Ralph was still here.

Again that night I shivered in the cold room, again I woke frequently to look at Ralph and listen to his breathing. Every now and then I heard him sigh.

In the morning I woke at 7:00 (thirty-four hours now) and went downstairs for a quick breakfast. I was somehow certain he would not die while I was out of the room. The nurse was there when I returned and suggested he might be more comfortable if the machines were turned off. "It's easier," she said.

"I'll call my kids in a little while. I want their opinions," I told her, but I knew the nurse was right. What good were machines now?

I read while the nurse finished up, then moved to sit beside the bed and hold on to Ralph. Words wouldn't come, but I wanted him to feel my touch.

A little past 9:00 his IV monitor beeped, and I rang for the nurse. As she came in, I moved and turned aside so she could get by.

After a few moments, I heard her gasp. "He's stopped breathing."

I turned back to Ralph.

He was gone.

CHAPTER 29

I expected this, readied myself for the final moments, but "ready" is only a word, not a state of mind. I saw everything through a gauzy cotton cloth, a screen that floated between me and reality. I wasn't sure I comprehended what happened. Was it some sort of convoluted dream?

People might ask, how can you be in shock when death is expected? You cleaned out the closets, contacted a funeral home. How much more grounded in reality can you be?

But no matter if you know the end is coming, no matter if you've rehearsed that moment a thousand times, until that final heartbeat, until that instant when your loved one is no longer warm and breathing by your side, no longer reachable, you don't really know. Loss is like pain; you can imagine it, but until it's real, you don't know how it feels. You can predict, you can visualize, believe you're ready but still be shocked and shaken when you face reality.

What I felt was a mixture of pain, like a piece of my heart had been sliced away, and disbelief: this couldn't be happening. In a moment, I'd blink and wake up. Despite this, the day was strangely ordinary. My body moved, I answered questions, remembered phone numbers.

I was no longer a wife, not yet truly a widow. I existed for the next hours in some sort of Neverland with its own rules, its own emotions and expectations.

I glanced at the clock. 9:10. Ralph had lived thirty-six hours and ten minutes, twelve plus hours longer than Dr. Helm had predicted. I think Ralph would have been pleased that he'd beaten her timetable.

He'd accepted his fate, left this life gently, died with dignity. Now I had to face the loss with equal dignity.

The nurse put her arms around me. Her eyes filled with tears. "He's at peace now," she said softly.

I hoped so. I hoped his religion would carry him safely to the other side, across the bar, to wherever good souls belong. There would be so many things to think of, to plan for, but now

I could only put one foot in front of the other, shuffle from one task to the next. I was standing at the precipice of the future, but I couldn't see beyond the first step. Not now, in the maelstrom of sorrow and anguish threatening to tow me under.

Tearfully I phoned my children, Ralph's sister and several close friends. I checked through Ralph's room. I was glad I'd cleaned out the closet and drawers days before. All that remained were his coin holder and a list of phone numbers. I put them in my bag.

While I waited for the chaplain, I watched Ralph. His chest seemed to move as it always had, but I knew that was my imagination. The doctor had already come in and pronounced him dead. His life was officially over.

Mine would go on in some fashion as I crossed the abyss I'd been dreading, the deep chasm between married life and widowhood.

The chaplain arrived. Lisa, the Jewish chaplain, was not there that day, but facing a stranger seemed somehow easier. We had no memories to share, no tears to shed together. We talked for a few minutes, and then he left.

Lori and Michael arrived to take one last look at the man who had been their surrogate father.

I kept my promise to Lori. I did not make a scene. Anyhow, I'd done that seven weeks earlier when the doctor said the leukemia returned and I'd shoved the staring lady out of the family room.

The nurse peeked in. I could tell she was anxious to prepare the room for its next occupant. One man's life was over; some other man, or woman, would take on their own battle in the place where Ralph had lost his.

My children left the room so I could have one more private moment with Ralph. I whispered my goodbye and kissed his forehead, and then I walked out and shut the door.

How strange to notice the staff going on about their morning duties as if nothing momentous had happened. I suppose a death isn't much of an event in a cancer hospital.

I walked outside past the rose garden and into the parking garage. How strange to get into my car and drive out of Garage 2 for the last time.

We went to Lori's, I made some more phone calls, and then we went to Jason's Deli for a quick lunch. The Sunday crowd chattered around us; yet I felt as if we were inside a bubble where nothing could reach us. After lunch Michael went home, Lori left to run an errand, and I lay down on her bed. Dazed, I tried to make sense of what had happened. I didn't feel pain or grief or much of anything. I just felt numb.

When Lori returned, she packed a few things for the night and we went to my house. There were messages on the answering machine, and for the rest of the evening the phone rang incessantly. I appreciated the expressions of sympathy, but talking to the many callers was exhausting.

Dana, a teacher from the synagogue school, called about a conference scheduled for the next afternoon. "My business partner is canceling it," I said. "My husband died this morning." The words came out as if I'd been rehearsing them all along. I guess I had.

Finally the phone stopped ringing, and Lori and I went to bed. Thanks to Ambien, I slept through the night.

The next morning felt odd, opening my eyes to a sunny fall day with no hospital visit to look forward to. No more visits ever again.

I was used to waking alone. I'd been by myself for seven months. But this was different. The path ahead was hidden, as if beyond a curve. The present was filled with plans to make – date and time of the funeral, airline reservations, a trip to the attorney's office to begin the probate process. Like others who have lost loved ones, I found the plans a way to get through the day, something to keep me energized, a means of stilling the thoughts and questions rolling around in my mind.

Some questions were unanswerable. What were Ralph's last thoughts? Where was he now – somewhere, nowhere? Other questions were more mundane. Did I need to buy a new shirt for him for the funeral? Jews are placed in their coffins in simple white shrouds; Christians wear regular clothes. For me, the questions from the funeral home were strange. For example, do you want your loved one to wear shoes? I decided I didn't.

That day and the rest of the week, there were two me's: the busy one and the still one, watching the other from inside herself, insulated, anesthetized, the me the outside world couldn't touch.

Ralph's sister Kate called and asked me to send pictures for a video to be shown at the funeral. I didn't want to. I told her I didn't have time, but Michael offered to e-mail her the pictures, so I selected a few, even though the idea of a video was strange to me. It wasn't what I was used to. Jewish funerals are austere. No flowers, no pictures, no music. Just the chant of Hebrew prayers and a plain wooden casket, always closed. I wondered if I would be able to bear the sight of an open casket. I discussed it with Dr. Payne. "I don't want to look," I said, and she assured me that I could do exactly what I chose. Still, I worried all week about the "viewing" and the video.

I needn't have. The video was charming, with pictures of Ralph as a child, a young man, and later with our family. His senior year picture from high school was included. The day before the funeral when we arrived at my mother-in-law's home, Lori noticed the blank space in the row of high school pictures and whispered to me with horror, "Mom, they took Ralph's picture down." In fact, they'd taken it to the funeral home to be used in the video.

The film ended with a picture of Tiki, Ralph's cat, perched on his TV.

I managed the viewing better than I expected. The family was allowed in first, and my mother-in-law took my arm and led me to the coffin. "No," I said, jerking away and went to sit with Lori. But later I had no choice. As friends filed past, the family was seated directly in front of the open casket. I lifted my eyes and looked at Ralph. I was surprised. All the horrors of cancer had been erased, and he looked like his old self, a healthy man, peacefully slumbering. I felt both relief and joy to be able to remember him like this.

And I was happy to be able to give his family the peace they needed. Ralph's funeral was a testament to their faith, and I was glad for it. If Ralph had not become ill, if he had not anticipated his death, I'm certain he would not have returned to his Christian faith. Therefore the leukemia, for all its tragedy, was, I supposed, a blessing. It restored his faith and assured him of heaven.

CHAPTER 30

When we returned to Houston, Lori dropped me off at my house. Suddenly I was alone. It was twilight, and the house was still. My future stared me in the face: evenings of loneliness to come.

Well, I told myself, I'd lost my husband, but I hadn't lost his voice. His greeting was still on our answering machine, saying in a flat, Midwestern twang, "You have reached the Zirkelbachs. Please leave a message at the sound of the tone. Thank you."

I promised myself I'd keep his greeting there. There were practical reasons. It's safer to have a man answer the phone. But the paramount reason was that hearing his voice was the closest I could be to him.

I sank down in a living room chair – Ralph's chair. I could almost smell his scent there. My spirits sinking along with my body, I glanced around the darkening room.

No! I wouldn't begin my widowhood by sitting and feeling sorry for myself. There was a memorial service to plan. I had given the Zirkelbachs the gift of a funeral in their faith; now it was time to plan a service in mine. I got up. It was early enough to call the rabbi to make arrangements.

I picked up the phone. There was no dial tone. I tried another phone. It was dead. I tried all six of our phones. None of them worked.

If the phone was dead, Ralph's voice was gone. I began to cry. I called Lori on my cell. She had no suggestions. I wandered into Ralph's study and stared at the console, pushed button after button to no avail. Could this have happened at a worse time? I'd buried my husband and now the last vestige of him was as unreachable as his body.

I sank down and rested my head on the desk. My gaze traveled to the floor.

And there I saw the telephone cord. Unplugged. The housekeeper must have knocked it out of the socket when she vacuumed the floor.

I plugged it in. There I raced into the family room and

grabbed my cell. Holding my breath, I dialed our number. The answering machine picked up. "You have reached ..."

Laughing with relief, I called Lori. "Guess what. I fixed it."

"How?"

I giggled. "I plugged it in."

Lori laughed, too. "Your first technological triumph."

The next days were busy, with the memorial service to plan. It took place on November 6. The synagogue's chapel was filled with friends, Ralph's business associates and mine. Friends came from Dallas, Valerie flew in from Connecticut. Many of the teachers at the school were there. Some didn't know him well, but the rabbi made sure, that by the time the service was over, they did. He spoke of his visits with Ralph and about our life together. He told funny stories about our first date to see "The Shoes of the Fisherman." He'd even gone to the trouble of looking up the movie and mentioned the stars and the plot. He talked about our family, our trips, our plans for the future.

Michael read a letter he had written and not been able to bring himself to give Ralph before he died:

"Dear Ralph,

It is hard to express myself right now with spoken words as I tend to get very emotional when I come to visit. So I thought I would write you this letter.

Although I have called you by your first name all of my life, I have always seen you as my father. You were there for us from almost the beginning and stayed with us through all of our birthdays, special holidays, graduations, and every milestone in our lives. This has continued with Gabriella and Marco. You have taken the role of their one and only grandfather. They will never forget you for that. And neither will Monica and I.

I just wanted to thank you for helping me grow into the man, husband and father I am today. And for being a fine husband to my mom, father to me, Lori and Bryan, and grandfather to Gabriella and Marco. You have had a major impact on all our lives and we will always love you

and appreciate everything you have done for us.
    You asked if Gabriella would remember you.
    I don't see how she could ever forget you.
    None of us will.
    Thanks for everything Dad, Grandpa.

    Love, Michael"

After the service and the speeches, we gathered at my house to share memories of Ralph. Some made us cry, others brought laughter. Penny, who began as my colleague and became a treasured friend to both of us, wiped away tears as she talked about the wonderful relationship Ralph and I had. She chuckled as she reminisced about a wedding the three of us attended in Galveston. On the way, the oil seal in our Volvo broke. "Did he insist on turning around and forgetting the wedding? No," she said. "He bought oil at a service station and every few minutes he stopped and added some. By the time we got home, he'd put in eighteen quarts. Now that's devotion."

Annette, a member of my writing group, recalled Ralph's love of chili peppers. She often sent him peppers from her garden. Rita remembered Ralph's kindness to her family when her grandson had problems several years before.

When everyone left, our family sat in the living room, tired and sad but gratified that so many had come to affirm their friendship with Ralph. We teased Bryan because so many of the female guests had remarked about how handsome he was. "You could be on the cover of one of your mom's books," one said, and Bryan flushed crimson with embarrassment.

Valerie gave me a small wooden box with a tile on the top picturing a pair of Sabbath candles and a scene of Jerusalem. "It's a memory box for you to fill," she explained. Over the next few weeks I put in a note written to Ralph by Gabriella on his sixty-fifth birthday; his pen which, in typical geek fashion, he'd always carried in his shirt pocket; his glasses, a business card, a tiny penguin as a souvenir of our trip to Antarctica, his recipe for turkey dressing, and a can of cat food as a reminder of his beloved Hal.

The memory box and a book of daily meditations called

Healing After Loss, which was sent by a colleague who'd recently lost her partner, were the two most loving gifts anyone gave me. And there were letters and cards. Peg Bartlett, owner of a frame shop and one of Ralph's favorite clients sent a card with a note that said, "We miss him, too." Jody Martin, a writing buddy of mine who had become friendly with Ralph, sent a note, mentioning that she'd once asked Ralph what he thought about when he wasn't working. "I solve problems in my head," he told her. It was a typical Ralph remark and the story made me laugh ... and cry.

When the weekend was over, the house cleared, Valerie on her way home, I woke to a Monday morning and took my first steps into the future.

CHAPTER 31

A year has passed since Ralph left my life. It's fall again, those crisp, bright days that will always remind of him. The time has gone by with the speed of a dream. Much of my life is unchanged. I live in the same house, although I've refurbished a bit, with a new fence, a flower garden behind the dressing room, and a new couch and chair in what used to be the junk room. I sleep in the same bed, still on "my" side; I've never thought of spreading out in the middle. My kitties sleep at the foot, Toby on the left, Tiki on the right. I moved Ralph's clothes out of my closet, except for his old brown bathrobe, which hangs on the hook where it always has. I haven't given his clothes away. Maybe someday. His voice is still on the answering machine, and the Monster, his philodendron, still dominates the patio. I have kept my promise not to cut it down.

But there are differences, too. Death is change. It causes a ripple effect that touches all aspects of the survivor's life.

My business partner Karlene and I closed our office at the end of May. I couldn't have dealt with discarding, packing, reviewing files the year before while Ralph was so ill. But as I hefted bags of materials I wanted to keep, carted them downstairs and later dragged them into my house, I realized how much easier the closing would have been with Ralph to help me with the heavy work.

A few days before our lease ran out, Karlene and I sat in the empty waiting room. "We've had lots of success," she said, "and we've always maintained our integrity."

I thought I would miss the office, but I haven't. I still work, seeing children at the private schools I've always served, but not as much as I used to. Just enough.

When Monica and Michael told their son Marco that Ralph had died, his first response was, "What will Thelma do when something breaks down?"

Cry.

After the tears, I began developing a support system: my

attorney, of course, a new accountant, a financial advisor, a handyman, an air conditioning technician. I didn't know Ralph's guys well and I frankly didn't like some of them, so I managed to find people I could depend on and who would work well for me. I wanted a business relationship, not the "I'll do you a favor and stop by when I have time" arrangement that Ralph had.

I even found a wonderful computer specialist who answered my desperate call the night before Thanksgiving when my hard drive crashed. Although he didn't save the hard drive, he made me feel better.

I long for Ralph when I need something minor done, something that seemed inconsequential when he was here to do it: unscrewing a tightly closed jar, getting down something for a high shelf, changing a light bulb in our high living room ceiling.

One day my smoke alarm began beeping to let me know its battery was dead. I couldn't reach it, not even with a ladder. Would my nerves survive listening to that annoying chirp for twenty-four hours until my housekeeper, who is taller than I am, could change the battery? No, I decided, and marched across the street and knocked on the door of the house directly opposite mine. Burdened with Ralph's illness, I'd never met the family who'd moved in there a year ago, but I'd seen the wife and I knew she was tall. I rang the bell, introduced myself, and explained my problem. Graciously, she followed me across the street and into my bedroom and quickly changed the battery. Problem solved.

Other things that are hard: moving heavy boxes, opening the safe in the garage, and especially, fastening necklaces. Oh yes, and dealing with bugs. Suzanne, my best friend in high school, still remembers my shrieks when a bug flew into the car.

I hate bugs, but I hate killing them even more. In Texas huge cockroaches often crawl in uninvited, even when the house has been sprayed. Ralph always dispatched them, but now it is my job. One night I glanced up and spied the biggest roach I'd ever seen ambling across the ceiling. I managed to get it down by tossing a box at it. Unwilling to squash it and deal with the aftermath, I doused it with bug spray as I followed it into the hall. Ten minutes later Tiki pounced at something. The roach. I sprayed it again, put a newspaper over it and decided I'd dispose of the remains in the morning. Within minutes it emerged from under the paper. I sprayed it again; it reappeared. Several dousings later, it finally expired. As I breathed a sigh and went back to bed, I decided the bug must have been a reincarnation of Rasputin, the Mad Monk of Russian fame, who was assassinated but had to be shot, strangled, and drowned before he succumbed.

But a bug was the least of my problems. One night I awoke to the sound of breaking glass. I figured the cats had knocked something down and got out of bed to investigate. Toby was in the living room, dozing on Ralph's chair; I found Tiki in the bathroom, but as I glanced in, I noticed her tail swishing wildly as she stared at the counter. I followed her gaze and spied something gray. Another cat?

I grabbed Tiki, shut the bathroom door, shooed her away, and then peeked in. Sitting on my counter, staring placidly at me was the most enormous possum I'd ever seen. We eyed each other like members of two rival gangs: the Jets and the Possums. What to do? Certainly not go in and confront the menacing marsupial, not with its sharp teeth. Try to chase it out into the garden? Same problem. I slammed the bathroom door.

I wanted Ralph here. Right now. But I reminded myself that he wouldn't have been any more able to deal with a wild animal than I was, and with that thought I went back to sleep. Near morning I began calling the SPCA, the Humane Society, every place I could think of. It was Labor Day weekend, the worst possible time to get help. Finally I called a private company. By the time they arrived, the possum had disappeared. "I'm not crazy," I told the young man. "I know there's a possum in here."

They found it hiding in a bag in my closet and took it away. Several days later they returned and animal-proofed the attic. The possum had come in that way, pushed down the attic stairs and made himself at home.

Besides the uninvited wild guests, I have endured two surgeries (a carpal tunnel release and a hysterectomy), a fall in the middle of the night that required a trip to the ER for stitches (I drove myself) a leaking air conditioner, a gas leak in the line from my hot water heater, and worst of all, the crash of my hard drive.

I have spent special days alone – New Year's Eve, Ralph's birthday, Valentine's Day – mourning for the one person who'd always been at my side.

I joined a grief group soon after Ralph died and found support and solace in the company of others who had loved and lost. One evening the group leader told us that we were blessed to have loved someone enough to mourn them. His statement turned grief on its head. How tragic it must be *not* to have someone to grieve.

I have become "more Jewish" during my widowhood. When I was a child, Judaism was part of the background of my life, like the Muzak you hear in elevators but don't really listen to. But now religion has moved to the forefront. Is it because I'm older and closer to death myself or that loss has led me to search more deeply for spirituality? I don't know the answer yet. But I am grateful for the strength my faith has given me because I have needed it to bear the bleak times ... and to celebrate the joyous ones. Yes, in spite of loss, I have still found joy in living.

Along with the pain of parting, I remember happy days with Ralph: good and sometimes not so good-natured political debates, listening to "A Prairie Home Companion" as we drove along a highway, sharing Thanksgiving with our children and their children, walking along a beach in Cozumel just before dawn. I remember one night glancing at the TV after I'd removed my glasses, noticing a blur of pink and remaking, "Look at those dancing girls."

"Put your glasses back on," Ralph said.

"Oh, my gosh." Not dancing girls, but flamingos. Several days later two garish pink plaster flamingos appeared in our back yard. Even for Ralph, the gaudy birds were too tacky for the front lawn.

Nearly thirty-five years of memories. Moments I took for granted.

In Thornton Wilder's "Our Town," after her death, Emily, the heroine, is given one day to relive. It's an ordinary day, but knowing now how significant, how precious is every moment of one's life, Emily cries out to her parents, "Can't we just *look* at each other?" Alas, they don't hear, and none of us do. If I could have one day to live over with Ralph ... but I can't. And even if I did, would I embrace the miracle of every ordinary moment? Perhaps, knowing what I do now, I would.

Grief is a puzzle. It comes and goes, washing over me at unexpected moments. Going through a file, I come across Ralph's handwriting on a sheet of paper and start to cry. Sometimes I sit on the couch that looks out onto my garden, reading a book, cuddled under Ralph's old brown robe. On New Year's Eve at midnight, I dialed our phone number to hear his voice on the answering machine so that, in some way, we could welcome the New Year together.

Never fond of poetry, in this year I have become a voracious reader, feasting on poems, welcoming the light they shed into the soul, and I have come to believe, with Wendell Berry, "that the dark, too, blooms and sings."

As I promised, I returned to Iowa in October. The leaves this year were not as bright, the wind sharper. As we drove through the town, Kate and Sara reminisced about Ralph's childhood. Kate remembered the day she and Ralph thought they'd unearthed an Indian burial ground behind their house and dug up the back yard searching for bones and how angry their father had been when he discovered them. I could picture Ralph as a gangly kid, with sweat running down his back as he wielded that shovel.

We drove to the cemetery and parked near Ralph's grave. The headstone I had ordered stood near his father's. Across the road I could see a field of corn, pale yellow stalks ready to be harvested. I'd brought Lori's digital camera so I could take a picture. I wanted the children to see his resting place, too.

The camera wouldn't work. I pressed buttons to no avail. *Dammit, Ralph*, I thought. *Fixing things was your job.*

"Give it to me," Kate said. She fiddled with it and handed it back.

I snapped the picture, checked the screen. Perfect.

I thought of Ralph's sister Sara singing "Amazing Grace" at

his funeral: "'Tis grace will lead me home." This was where Ralph belonged, in the home of his childhood, in the bosom of his Lord. The abandonment I felt when he told me he had returned to Christianity disappeared, swept away on that windy afternoon. I placed a pebble on the headstone, a Jewish custom when one visits a grave. It shows that someone has honored and remembered the dead and unlike flowers, which wither, stones last forever.

I promised Ralph I'd be back when another year has come and gone.

I will.

CPSIA information can be obtained at www.ICGtesting.com
Printed in the USA
BVOW040849180313

315595BV00002B/7/P